D1496305

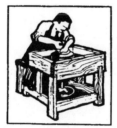

TM

By the same author:

Through Hells Gates to Shanghai, Lawhead Press, 1983

It Began at Imphal, Sunflower University Press, 1987

Never A Ho-Hum Day, An Autobiography

Doc, My Tiger's Got An Itch

The True Story of a Kentucky Hill Country
Veterinarian Who Occasionally Runs Away
With The Circus.

by

JOHN G. MARTIN, DVM

With Introduction by
Gee Gee Engesser

Guild Press of Indiana
Indianapolis, Indiana 46228

ISBN 1-878208-87-X

CONTENTS

INTRODUCTION

In the early 1960s I presented a sled dog act—THE ALASKANS. One of my star canine performers got sick; and, on the suggestion of another performer, I called veterinarian Dr. John Martin to help me. Without a minute's hesitation, he left his home late at night to attend my malamute. He came with no regard for time of day to help me and demonstrate his compassion for his animal patient. He helped my dog, and this was the beginning of a lasting friendship.

His wife Mary Helen, through her childhood friendship with Ernestine Clarke Baer, lighted the spark that started "Doc" on his way to being a circus veterinarian. His first circus work started with the Mills Brothers Circus working for Jack, Jake and Harry. When the Mills show took down its Big Top for the last time, Dr. Martin moved on to Sells & Gray, Clyde Brothers Circus, Ringling Bros. and Barnum & Bailey Circus and smaller shows with such titles as Clark & Walters and Fisher Brothers Circus. His reputation as a circus veterinarian was made with his sincere interest in developing state-of-the-art exotic animal medicine fortified by his compassion for the circus, its animals and their owners. His reputation grew, and it didn't take long for most of the animal acts and circuses to call for his services.

Determined to be a good circus doctor, he asked for animal handling tips and help from such greats as Charlie Moroski—one of the all time great horse trainers, Hugo Schmidt, Ringling's superintendent of elephants, Colonel Trevor Bale, Charly Baumann and Robert Baudy.

Dr. J. Y. Henderson, Ringling Bros. and Barnum & Bailey Circus Staff Veterinarian, soon saw Dr. Martin's potential and guided him down the sawdust trail. Together they were the pioneers of circus veterinary medicine. They developed new surgical techniques and medical ideas that saved many circus animal's lives.

It didn't take long for most of the good animal trainers—Jack Joyce, Karley Peterson, Bucky Steele, Wally Naughton, Andrew

Kirby the chimp man, Bobby Gibbs—and many other animal people to realize that Dr. Martin was sincere with his desire, and talented with his ability to be a healer of our kind of animals.

As the years went by, "Doc" and his wife Mary Helen became very dear personal friends of me and my family. Their daughter Terri trouped with us on the Clyde Brothers Circus in '65. She affectionately earned the name of "Cotton Candy Queen" working for me and my husband in the "floss" joint.

This is Dr. Martin's story. This book relates just a few of the things that happen in a career like his in the atmosphere of the Big Top and show business. It tells of the heartbreak, the hardships, the funny and not so funny things on the circus lot or in the buildings.

Like many of the animal act owners and show owners, I appreciate knowing and working with Dr. Martin. He has never hesitated to help any of us when we call him to consult or prescribe for or surgically attend our animals.

Most of us in the world of the circus are born into it. A very few others earn their way to the inside and become one of us. Doc Martin is one of those few —he earned it. He is truly a circus veterinarian—he is part of today's circus!

We in the performing animal world applaud him.

Gee Gee Engesser

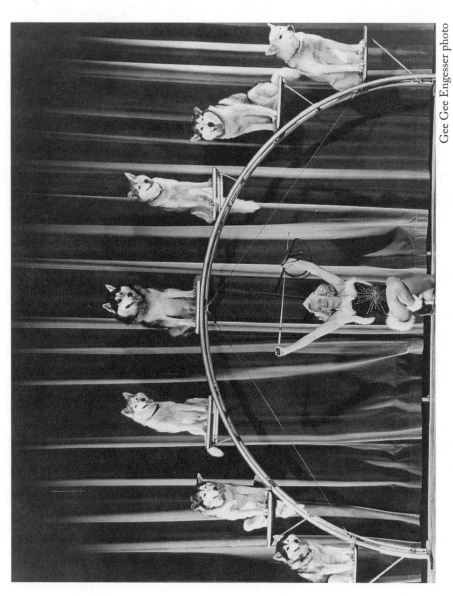

Gee Gee Engesser and The Alaskans. Gee Gee is an outstanding performer and show producer, truly a grand lady of the circus.

Gee Gee Engesser photo

THE COME-IN

The "Come-In" in circus talk is the time when the audience enters the Big Top, or arena, just before the show begins. Most generally a performer, usually a clown, entertains the audience, exciting them and stimulating their imagination about the circus. Besides being entertaining, this is a hint of what is to come. It prepares the audience for the big show. Call this, if you want, my Come-In.

When I was nine years old, in 1933, my parents sent me from our home in Portsmouth, Ohio, to Ashland, Kentucky, to visit my grandparents. I was their first grandchild and I must have been very special to them. While I was with them they spent their waking hours entertaining me and showing me off to their friends. Maybe it was fate, or maybe just by chance, during this visit the timing was just right—a circus was coming to town!

The circus advance man and the show's bill posters did their work well. Ashland's buildings, fences and store windows were covered with posters from the Hagenbeck-Wallace Circus. Farmer's barns and abandoned buildings were all decorated with these gaudy advertisements. Most of the brightly colored paper showed a young lion tamer named Clyde Beatty cracking his whip in the face of a ferocious lion! The circus advertising men, with their hoopla, were successful and nearly everyone was waiting for the "Big Show"—as the posters advertised—to come to town.

My grandpa, grandma and my Uncle Fred took me to the circus. With Grandpa holding one of my hands and grandmother the other, we followed my uncle as he guided us through the crowded midway toward the main entrance. Candy butchers hawked their wares, and as we passed the gaily painted banners advertising the freaks and oddities along the bally line of the side show, a pitch man, called a talker, expounded on the sights to be seen inside his tent. His spiel rang out, "Just for ten cents—only one tenth of a dollar—come see the side show." Lines of people, dimes in hand, pushed to the ticket seller, eager to see what was hidden behind the side walls of canvas.

The huge canvas Big Top was filled with people. It was hot and dusty and all of the mysterious smells of the circus permeated the tent. We found our seats, the circus band blared a lively tune and the show started. All of the performers, horses, camels and elephants paraded around the hippodrome track. The spectators applauded loudly at this amazing sight.

The large steel arena was set up in the center ring, and as the last of the performers and the animals paraded out of the big tent, the ringmaster blew his whistle and directed everyone's attention to the center ring when he said in a loud, resonating voice, "Ladies and gentlemen, directing your attention to the steel arena, Hagenbeck-Wallace Circus proudly presents—the master of the wild beasts!" (He paused to let his description fill every ear.) "The world's youngest lion and tiger trainer," (he paused again to get the crowd's attention,) "Mr. Clyde Beatty!" A huge roar of approval filled the Big Top as Mr. Beatty, whips and chair in hand, entered the large cage and signaled his helper to let the first cat in.

Tigers and lions came into the arena and one by one, under Beatty's directions, mounted the pedestals. The act went on, Beatty cracking the whip, shooting his blank pistol and shouting commands. The crowd applauded with every new trick. Then—quick as a flash, a tiger jumped from its high stand to the back of another tiger on a lower pedestal and with claws and teeth, ripped the skin from the victim's shoulder making a long jagged cut about ten inches long!

The fighting tigers were vicious—tearing at each other with teeth and claws, roaring and screaming in their lust to kill. Tiger blood and saliva were everywhere. It was utter chaos. Cage men added more to the confusion and excitement as they prodded the tigers with long poles through the bars of the arena trying to break up the fight. In the middle of the big cage, almost clouded by the dust of the fight, Clyde Beatty, cracking his whip and shooting his pistol, was seemingly in control of the situation. One by one he herded all of the big cats except the wounded tiger into the chute and back to their cage wagons. The fight was over.

As the spellbound audience watched, Beatty managed to get a lasso rope around the tiger's neck and with the help of his assistants, pulled the ailing cat up to the bars of the cage. Then someone reached through the bars and poured what appeared to be iodine all over the wound! The tiger roared and screamed—no doubt in shock and unquestionably in pain. Circus veterinary medicine—such as it was at that time—was done. The cat was turned loose and in a flash he headed for the tunnel and his own domain! The crowd cheered their approval. Mr. Clyde Beatty took his accolades as if nothing unusual had happened. The ringmaster blew his whistle to announce a new act, and in that hot crowded Big Top, the show went on!

That was the last year that Clyde Beatty was with the Hagenbeck-Wallace Circus. He left the circus in 1934 to form his own show, the Cole Brothers & Clyde Beatty Circus. I grew older and Mr. Beatty is gone, but I will never forget that day. Now, looking back, I wonder if it might have had some bearing on my future.

But before I had grown up to be nine years old and saw Mr. Beatty, young master of the lions and tigers, do his work, there were other little things that surely influenced my later life.

One day when I was about five years old, my mother tied me to the front porch with a clothes line rope. I had to have been embarrassed but there I was, a runaway—paying the penalty for my latest adventure. This time I had gone up Sinton to Gallia Street, then around the corner past Henry's Tavern to my favorite observation post, the curbstone in front of Mr. Hicks' grocery store. When I got the chance, I would sit there spellbound, watching my small world of wonders. It was an exciting time for a youngster my age. It was a time of inventions and new ideas. I can remember watching one of our lady citizens drive down the street in her almost silent electric car. Clattering behind her, usually impatient with her snail-like pace, were frustrated drivers of the noisier A and T model Fords. On very rare occasions, a tiny airplane droned through the sky and, like nearly everybody in 1929, I would look up and stare at that marvel too. Across the street from the grocery, in front of the shoe factory, was a watering trough for horses. It was one of three still left in my home town. I remember one time sitting on my curbstone perch, watching the milk man guide his horse to the trough for a drink. The driver stepped down from his wagon, pulled a big red bandanna from his pocket, and wiped the sweat from his forehead, while he waited patiently for his horse to satisfy his thirst. A cloud of English sparrows fluttered down from a shoe factory window ledge to the dusty road at the horse's feet. The horse, switching its tail to scatter the flies and the aggravating little brown birds, drank its fill and was again ready to serve his master. That's all I remember about the horse that day, but I have never forgotten my mother, who after a frantic search, found me and then tethered me to the porch so it wouldn't happen again.

I was entranced with that horse, and every time I heard it, I ran to the street and watched it plod by. What magic does a horse hold for some people? Most kids, especially boys, are fascinated by horses and nearly every kid in my time dreamed of owning a pony. A lot of youngsters dreamed about ponies and horses, but few in my generation, in the heart of the Great Depression, ever had the chance to feed and care for one of their own.

Those old water troughs, like the horse-drawn delivery wagons, are gone, having no place now in today's world. But horses are not gone and the fascination for them is not gone either. Some call this attraction "horse fever." I have been afflicted with it all of my life.

One hot summer day—it had to be in 1929—the circus came to my home town. My daddy and my mother tended me this time in front of Mr. Hicks' grocery as the circus paraded by my special place. Best I can recall, it was the Sells-Floto Circus.

Great parade wagons pulled by Percheron Horses, their gray

coats dappled with darker spots, creaked along the street—proud drivers expertly handling their teams. Clowns brought laughs with their painted faces. Uniformed musicians riding high on top of the richly carved and gilded band wagon filled the air with brassy marching tunes. The elephants shuffled along the hot pavement, and fancy high stepping riding horses stirred up the street dust. They captivated young and old alike. And then, the very last wagon rolled by, belching steam from its pipes and filling the air with the loud boisterous music of the calliope. As the calliope signaled the end of the parade, the street watchers fell in behind it and, like rats following the piper, followed the parade to the circus lot. Today those circus parades are like ghosts—something out of the past, never to happen again. I'm glad I saw those days. The tented circus was in its heyday, a real part of Americana. A young person like me couldn't help but be absolutely fascinated by it all, especially by the horses!

Those fancy circus horses, and no doubt the horse that pulled the old milk wagon, played a part in my destiny as a veterinarian and what has since proved to be a most interesting life.

In the late twenties my home town, like the rest of America, was in the grips of the Great Depression. Besides this, parents of many kids my age had just been through the horrors of World War I. The scars of both were evident. These were unsettled times. But we were progressing. Most folks had radios and telephones in their homes. Franklin Roosevelt, our newest President, promised prosperity and salvation when he created the WPA, the PWA and other initial-designated organizations. To a kid of six, who cared? Horses and ponies and the smell of horse sweat fascinated me. Most everybody was fascinated by airplanes. "Lucky Lindy" Lindbergh, just a short time before, had flown his airplane, the Spirit Of St. Louis, to France and was number one on the hero list. Some of the kids' fathers had been pilots who flew the flimsy fighters over France during the war. The stories these men told held everyone spellbound. Never mind, I still wanted a pony and the answer was always the same, "We can't afford it—where would you keep it?" I heard that song sung many times before I had my first honest-to-goodness live horse.

President Roosevelt's WPA, NRA and the other A's worked, and slowly America dug its way out of the depression into another era. It was called the "thirties." Kids my age were growing up in a new kind of society. Lifestyles were rapidly changing and most families now owned an automobile which they proudly parked in the old carriage house or stable. The horse had had it. The gasoline engine did him in. I still wanted a pony.

My father was a civil engineer and through the depression was fortunate enough to have a job. It was with the WPA. As times got better, he and mother had a house built out at the edge of town. I grew up in that house and by this time, being seven or eight years old, I could see that we now had the place for the pony. But we still could not, what with a new baby brother, ". . . afford it." At that young age I figured a pony would be more fun.

My mother was a devoted housewife, catering to her husband and doting on her children. Growing up was not so hard. Like a lot of kids, I didn't care too much for school but I had to go. Instead of classrooms I would rather have roamed the woods and watched the quail and rabbits—they were plentiful then. It was more fun to take a long stick and poke it up into a hollow tree and scare the flying squirrels out of their dens into a waiting burlap bag or shoot at a robin with my Daisy BB Gun. I tried trapping rabbits with a box and a stick and a long string, using carrots for bait. I didn't catch any.

I remember my mother, on more than one occasion, trying to hustle me out the door so I wouldn't be late for class. Radio adventures fascinated me, and I usually lingered, hoping to hear Little Orphan Annie's dog Sandy broadcast his last "Arf" of the day on the Ovaltine radio show. Like most other boys my age, I was spellbound by Jack Armstrong, The All-American Boy, who expounded the merits of Wheaties. I was entranced by an early time country music singer by the name of Bradley Kincaid. I could just imagine him strumming his guitar and singing his theme song, "In The Hills Of Old Kentucky." I could see those hills from my house and after mother disenchanted me from radio station WPAY, I sometimes hummed that tune on my way down the hill to school.

I managed the grammar school and eventually I made it to high school. During all this time, my desire for a horse never let up. The subject came up nearly everyday. Finally Mother got interested and suggested to Father that maybe now. ". . . we could afford one." Father knew a local horse trader and after my dad conferred with him, the trader agreed to loan us a horse for the winter. He figured that was a good way to get it fed and cared for free. She was a sorrel mare with blazed face and two white stockings on her rear legs. The owner called her Annie Laurie. We made the arrangements, and after building an addition to the back of our garage, we brought her home and at last I had what I wanted—my own horse—even though we had borrowed it for just a short time.

Doctor Owen M. Karr was the local veterinarian. I knew him because we had taken our dogs to him for vaccinations and wormings. We visited his office, only three blocks away, when the dog got sick or needed shots or other care. With the acquisition of the horse, Dr. Karr became a frequent visitor to our house, tending Annie when she was not well. He soon became my idol, and at every opportunity I managed to visit his office. His skills with an animal soon had my complete attention. It was then that I knew I was going to be a veterinarian.

Annie Laurie stayed with us that winter, and finally in early spring we sent her back to her owner. By now the entire family had the horse fever. Father, now outvoted, bought a big pony for me and an old, smaller one for little brother. Mother found a pretty little easy-riding black mare. We were in the horse business. With three, we also saw Dr. Karr more often.

The last of the thirties saw me in the first grades of high school. I wore cowboy boots to class, and looking back at the times I feel sorry for those that sat close to me because I knew those boots always smelled like horse manure. All of my free time was spent with the horses. I rode one or the other all over the town. I visited my friends, went to the grocery and once even ducked my head and rode the pony into Mother's kitchen! For this Father did more than talk, even though I was high school size! I was indeed a knight, without armor, on my horse.

An era that became known as "the roaring forties" began. To me it meant senior high school and dates and dances—it was a real whirl. School in the winter and working for my father, who now owned an engineering company, in the summers kept me busy. One summer I worked for a big construction company. They specialized in earth construction projects. We built a levee along the river bank. Its purpose—to keep the flooding Ohio River out of our town. I helped the surveyor on that job. From one place along that levee I could see where my girlfriend, Mary Helen Feyler, worked. Sure enough, when we worked in that area, we could always see her standing at her office window waving at us. Her compassionate boss, Ben Cross, commented that if the town ever flooded again it would be at that low place we had worn in the flood wall while we courted. As a matter of interest, I later married that girl. These jobs took up the daylight hours, but at night I was always at the veterinary office of my friend Dr. Karr. He tolerated me and finally let me do some menial things around the office. I was grateful. On a few occasions he took me with him on his farm calls where he treated the larger animals. That was fun. I spent more and more time there and let it be known at home that someday I was going to be just like "Doc" Karr.

Nineteen thirties years were now history and the new decade was born, clouded by political unrest and the threat of another World War. America watched apprehensively. The future was unsure. Shortly before my graduation, my father talked to me about my plans for after high school. Without reservation, I told him I wanted to be a veterinarian. Looking me straight in the eye he hesitated and finally said, "Son, who in the hell ever heard of a cow doctor making a living?" He further added that he thought I should go to an engineering school since I had some idea of what that was all about. In the same breath he mentioned the fact that with war clouds nearly over us, I could probably get a deferment from the military, at least until I finished school. I protested but my weak argument bore no fruit. Father had committed me—I did not like it.

THE YOUNG YEARS, A WAR,
THE DREAM COMES TRUE

Mother packed my clothes, Father gave me a train ticket and a slide rule, and I headed towards Virginia to college. They were determined that I would become a surveyor of land and a builder of buildings.

The academic part of college was very hard for me. When it got too hard, I sneaked off to the college farm and watched the cows and the horses. With effort I managed to squeak by the chemistry, physics, drafting and calculus. Surveying classes were easier because I had learned something about that while working for my father. At the end of the year I pleaded with my father not to make me go back. Once more he said, "Son, you're headed the right way. Go back and finish." I again brought up the veterinary medicine subject but he was emphatic, saying "No."

I started my sophomore year thinking that Father had probably been right about becoming an engineer. I pursued it without enthusiasm. But the cannons of war were shaking the entire world and it was inevitable that sooner or later most of us would have to answer the call for military service. I had given that some thought too, but didn't know exactly what I was going to do.

One day, leaning over the farm fence watching a cow lick her calf, I heard an airplane, and up in the clouds another "Lucky Lindy" made the decision for me. I wanted to learn to fly. The day after Thanksgiving I left college and enlisted in the Army Air Corps Flying Cadet program. After I signed the papers and held up my hand for the swearing in, I called home and told my parents what I had done. Father was elated—Mother was crying—I was out of that school and civil engineering.

America's lifestyle, as everybody knows, was changed dramatically. Everybody but the physically disabled—the draft boards classified them "4-F"—was in uniform. Troop trains with shades drawn at night, going to secret destinations, crossed and recrossed our country. Women became riveters and welders and did other men's work too. The nation was in a frenzy of excitement. It was the greatest adventure most of us would ever have, but some would be wounded and disabled while many would pay the high price for glory with their lives. After months of rigorous training, I earned my silver pilot wings and my gold second lieutenant's bars. Eventually I learned to fly a cargo airplane, a C-47, and was sent to India. Our job was to support our fighting soldiers either by air dropping supplies, or landing in tiny jungle airstrips. I flew my missions with pride for my country and sometimes with pure fear in my heart. I saw the Far East, the Taj Mahal, the Indian Fakirs and their snakes. I saw it all, or better yet, all I wanted to see.

Some of the things we saw fit this story and bear telling. We departed Florida and flew down over the Caribbean to South America, across the ocean to Africa and from there eventually to Aden, a city in what is now known as Yemen. This was to be an overnight stop. Landing early in the afternoon and, after securing our billets for the night, we rode a GI truck into town to see the sights.

Aden is an ancient city perched on the beaches at the confluence of the Red Sea and the Gulf of Aden. The city's back doors rest at the foot of high hills which hold back the sands of the Arabian Desert. The sprawling city is drowned in sunshine the year around. It is a hot, dusty and dirty place. We walked up and down the streets, never missing anything. The dark skinned men wore long, loose, white robes and head pieces called a burnoose. The women all were dressed in long, loosely-fitting black dresses. The females also wore a scarf-like head piece, the bottom of which was always fastened over the lower part of their face like a veil. They in no way resembled the voluptuous beauties we saw in our movies. They were dirty and, by our standards, not very pretty. Of course it is said, ". . . that beauty is in the eyes of the beholder." The streets were crowded, noisy and filthy. We passed all kinds of shops and stores, each merchant holding his hand out trying for our Yankee dollars. It was pure fascination for us nineteen-year-old grownups. The butcher's store impressed me. His cuts of meat hung on hooks in front of his stall. Green flies swarmed over every piece. It almost turned my stomach and for sure it didn't resemble the spotlessly clean meat market down on Market Street back home in Ohio!

Walking farther we came to a new, modern, impressive building, an absolute contrast to the surrounding architecture. It was three stories tall, and leading to each level was a ramp about ten feet wide. We wondered what it could be. We couldn't read the sign because it was printed in Arabic. Our curiosity was soon solved as a dark skinned native man, robe and burnoose flapping, drove his limping camel up the ramp for treatment. This was a camel hospital! I stood there for several minutes, wondering what some Arabian veterinarian was going to do to that beast. Surely it would be interesting to work on these animals. At the time I didn't know how mean, despicable or ornery an old camel could get, but that is getting ahead of my story. Impressed by Asia's modern veterinary medical facility, we wandered back toward the truck and our ride to the airport. While we waited at the truck-stop for our vehicle, three Arabs, dressed just like the camel driver, rode by us on gray dappled horses. These had to be pure Arabian Horses—after all this is where they came from. The horses were thin and had sores on their legs and sides. Their eyes watered from fly bites in spite of the nets that hung down from the bridles. These animals were small and seemed undersized for those that rode them. The riders, looking nothing like movie star sheiks, galloped by, swirling the dust and flies before us. We didn't understand a thing they said and certainly we weren't impressed with their exhibition. The next day we flew on to India and more adventures.

India. It is a land beyond belief with all kinds of people, all kinds of religions, all kinds of climates and weather and all kinds of strange things—human or otherwise! The big cities and the little towns are all alike. India is like a jar full of tinkling bells, swarms of people, constant noise, disease and poverty. The sacred cattle roam freely through the streets of the towns, soiling, everything with their cow type of sanitation. No one seems to mind. The lepers and diseased lay in the ditches but the cattle were blessed. As an aspiring veterinarian, I wondered what kind of exotic diseases they might have.

Like most young men I was fascinated by the animals—the same ones that the circuses carried in their menageries. But instead of being tended by uniformed circus animal handlers, they were here in the jungles in abundance. Elephants roamed free in the jungle and sometimes coming home from our missions at night, the control tower operator would tell us to, ". . . and with caution, elephants are on the runway!" Tigers and other dangerous animals seemed to be behind every clump of jungle and the snake was ever-present.

We lived on an airfield close to the village of Sylhet. Sylhet is in what is now Bangladesh, just ten miles from Karapunji, the place reported to have the heaviest rainfall in the world. We lived in bamboo houses with thick grass roofs. These buildings were called bashas and were scattered along the jungle paths that meandered over the area of our airbase. We learned to use the mosquito netting over our beds at night and faithfully took our Atabrine tablets to prevent us from getting malaria. We also learned that it was wise to take the covers off the bed and remake it before you went to sleep just in case a snake had decided to make his home there in the daytime. It became routine to shake out our shoes before putting them on every morning to be sure that a scorpion had not found them a good hiding place! We tolerated the incessant rain of the monsoon and we soon accepted the fact that the surrounding jungle was home for exotic creatures like the cobra, the python and a small green snake, the krait.

Living on our jungle airbase was like living in a zoo. The trees were full of chattering monkeys busy raising their families and looking at us like we were intruders in their world. Clouds of brightly colored parrots and other exotic birds nested in the trees. At night jackals, the Indian leopard and tigers added their conversations to the constant noise of the jungle.

I never was a snake fancier and shuddered then—and to this day—at the mere thought of one. I have one vivid memory about our stay in Sylhet and the jungle creatures. I had flown my missions for the day and came home from the airstrip in the truck and climbed the hill to our basha. As I approached my bamboo and grass house, I saw several American enlisted men and some flying officers, plus our Indian houseboy, Joe Mia, standing in the path in front of the basha. Joe was wide eyed and jabbering half in English and half in Bengalese about a huge snake that he saw slither from a bamboo thicket in the jungle across the basha porch into the room that I lived in! I questioned Joe and he said, ". . . big snake, Sahib, big, big, big!" One of the enlisted men vouched for his statement as he had seen it too. We never did find that big snake, nor where he exited my bedroom. Needless to say, my roommates and I slept with apprehension that night. I am sure that the reptile entered the front door and without stopping, continued through the back wall to his jungle home. The snake was a large python. Sylhet was a different world, an exciting place during exciting times.

In 1945, my tour of combat duty was over and while still in India, I gathered my college credits from previous schooling and sent them to the Dean of Admissions, College of Veterinary Medicine at Ohio State University.

PLANNING FOR TOMORROW

It was three months since the *S.S. Exchequer* slipped past the Statue of Liberty into New York Harbor and disgorged her load of returning American soldiers. I came home on that ship and after a stint in a California hospital and a few days signing papers I became a civilian.

The summer of 1945 was a lazy time. I found a job doing the only thing I knew how to do—flying. I was hired as a flying instructor at our local airport. After flying all day my evenings were religiously devoted to Dr. Karr's veterinary hospital. I was more determined than ever to pursue that profession. What time was left was spent courting the girl that I wrote the letters to from India—the same one who waved at me when I worked on the flood wall, Mary Helen Feyler.

In the evenings, when my airport work was through, I drove straight to Dr. Karr's office. I stayed in the background and watched him do his magic. He taught me how to hold the pets while he looked at them, let me watch and would give me a complete description of each case and his decision as to treatment. He obviously was interested in me. After the last small animal patient left, we usually had one or two farm calls to make, and so off we would go to tend some ailing horse or cow or pig. I was impressed and more sure than ever I had made the right choice. I learned much from Dr. Karr that summer, and armed with his moral support, I applied for entrance to the Ohio State University for the fall semester.

Mary Helen and I discussed our plans. Our first decision was to get married. We would find a place to live in Columbus, I would go to college and get my degree as a Doctor of Veterinary Medicine and she would do what she could to help out. My God, you should have heard the fuss. My mother cried and insisted we just couldn't make it, being married and going to college at the same time. Mary Helen's mother chimed in with the same story. Mary Helen's father, a dental surgeon, gruffly said, "Let 'em alone. I have no doubts about either one of them." So that is where it stood. I went away to college for my pre-veterinary medicine educational requirements. We got married the day after Christmas, 1945.

Married life proved to be great, and together we sought a place to live. We found a tiny apartment close to the university. It had one room and a kitchen plus a share-the-bath with six male students. The sink leaked, there were cockroaches under the cabinets and the floors and the walls were filthy dirty, but it was a start. I patched the leaking sink, talked the landlord into buying some paint, and we went to work making it livable. Everything was great except we had no money other than what little I was entitled to as a veteran.

We both were determined to make it, and there was never any question that I would eventually do anything but practice veterinary medicine. After my pre-professional school requirements were finished, I applied for acceptance to the College of Veterinary Medicine. With Dr. Karr's recommendations, and other qualifications, I was accepted.

Sixty-two students were seated in the amphitheater of the veterinary college building. The building was old, and the wooden floors squeaked as you walked on them. Noises from other parts of the building filtered through the plastered walls and animal odors hung in the air. It had been very competitive getting there and all sixty-two were excited. Some introduced themselves to a neighbor; others silently waited for the session to begin.

At the foot of the tiered seats was a rostrum; behind that a door led to some unknown place. Precisely on the hour, a man stepped through the door and walked up to the rostrum. The silence was awesome. Hesitating briefly, he surveyed the sixty-two eager faces, and finally said, "Gentlemen, welcome to the Ohio State University

College of Veterinary Medicine. I am Dr. Walter Krill. I am the Dean of the College." His eyes scanned every face as if trying to fix each person in his mind. With these brief remarks, Dr. Krill opened the way for sixty-two of us to become Doctors of Veterinary Medicine.

The next four years were hard times, but, of course, rewarding. My wife worked and I worked a full time job besides going to school. No one ever gave us a cent—we made it on our own.

I am pleased that I got my education from the teachings of the old masters of veterinary education. I have often said I was one of the last to graduate from the old time "horse doctor" schools of veterinary medicine. I am grateful for this and give my sincere thanks to Drs. Grossman, Goss, Schaulk, Guard, Rudy, Cole, Tharp, Venzke and others who tutored the class of 1950.

There were ups and downs and hard times, but being married we faced them together—the good luck and the bad—the adventures and the not-so-glamorous.

There were some times I will never forget about college days. During my first year in "vet school," anatomy was our biggest class. Dr. James Grossman, the Almighty of Veterinary Anatomy, was our teacher. He wrote the text book we used and which is—now nearly 50 years later—still the Bible for animal muscles and bones.

The first animal we worked on was the horse. It was used as a basis of comparison with other animals. Old Dobbin made a good foundation. Every student had a horse skeleton of his own. Mine was stabled—when he wasn't in use—in a big box under our bed.

We dissected him piece by piece, learning the names of every bump, muscle, bone and blood vessel in the cadaver. We never had a day off from school, and we looked forward to Christmas and a little vacation with our families. The old cadaver was draped with formaldehyde soaked sheets and we wheeled him into his refrigerated stall for the school break. No one gave the horse another thought.

After the holidays were over, well endowed with presents, we took what we needed back to Columbus and crammed them all into our little one-room hovel. Among the gifts was a case of strawberry preserves my mother made especially for us. They were great. We needed all of the groceries we could get. I went back to school that first morning stuffed with home made biscuits that had been covered with mother's preserves. First class that day was anatomy lab. I met Lou Motyca and Dave Crill at the door and we went straight to the cold box to wheel out what was left of our cadaver. Dave opened the heavy door and walked in to roll the horse out. The two week respite from our crude surgery had allowed our specimen to grow a new coat—this one, a dull green coat of mold! That didn't bother us too much but once we got him rolled to our table and removed the form-aldehyde soaked sheets, that horse cadaver smelled exactly like Mother's strawberries! To this day, I just can't stomach strawberry preserves!

My first year in college was full of trials and tribulations. I had to learn all over how to study and how to learn. My new bride did more than her share, and we somehow managed to make ends meet. Happiness was our ups, and I guess that our apartments were our downs. Shortly after we fixed up our apartment, the landlord came to us and told us we would have to move! The reason? He could get more money by renting to single males. So out we went to find an-other place to live. Once more we painted and scrubbed and fixed and repaired. That one lasted only a short time too. Reason? Same thing, money and greed. We went through several one-roomers and even-tually rented a three-room apartment from a classmate. That one lasted, but not until we painted and scrubbed and repaired that place too.

Bill, my classmate, and Donna Bechdolt owned a house down on Indianola Avenue. Bill's father had financed the house for them. They lived downstairs. Upstairs was a three room and bath apartment. It was empty except for an old fashion ice box and a decrepit gas range. The front room had a gas heater; the kitchen was warmed by the cooking stove. The bedroom, sandwiched between the other two, got its heat from a hole cut through the floor above Bechdolt's dining room. Bill and Donna used the rent money to pay on the mortgage.

We didn't even inquire about the cost. We said, ". . . we'll take it . . . ."

Finally we got to be juniors in college. The new status had prestige and opened the way for actual participation in the sick animal business. Besides our lectures, we participated in the clinics. We went to lectures in the mornings and spent the afternoons and Saturday, plus Sunday mornings, in different wards of the veterinary clinic. It was hard work with long hours and little time for recreation. Most of the students were married and all of us suffered the same ailments—mostly lack of money and hard times. Many of the wives worked and most of the students had after-hours jobs to help pay the bills of living.

Entertainment was nearly nonexistent except what we could make for ourselves. On some weekends, Bill's father, who was a barber, and his mother would come to Columbus for a visit. They were from Wapakoneta, Ohio. Mr. Bechdolt was boisterous and, like his son, a great beer drinker. They brought with them some pork hearts, shrimp and a case of beer. We cooked the pork hearts in the pressure cooker with some pickling spices and soaked the shrimp in vinegar. This became ritual and the feast of the pork, beer and shrimp made a grand party.

There were other incidents too that added to our college experiences.

Across the street from our house we befriended our neighbors, the Fullers. They came to our Saturday night parties too. Glen Fuller worked in one of the factories and if his wife Gay didn't intercept him on payday, he would spend it all on beer. It was a race to see who got to spend the paycheck! Gay had been winning for some time and Glen was pretty well dried out. One Saturday evening, Bill and I were sitting on the front steps talking when Glen came over and wanted to know if we had any beer. We did, but we told him we didn't. We weren't selfish, just prudent, because we knew if he got into it, he would drink it all. He thought a minute and mentioned that he knew how to make beer out of potatoes. It sounded like a great idea and we agreed to buy the spuds if he would concoct the brew. We had a deal.

At the same time Glen mentioned a tom cat that was making our street his prowling grounds, fighting and breeding every cat in the neighborhood. He squalled and carried on all night. As a matter of fact, Mary Helen and I heard him sound off on more than one occasion. Bechdolt, in an off-hand manner, suggested that now that we were about to become veterinary surgeons, we should castrate him. Glen agreed and said he would bait the old cat onto his side porch so we could catch him. It was agreed. Next day Bill and I got out the surgery book and we read about how to neuter a tom. This was to be our very first surgery case and after studying the textbook, we considered ourselves ready for the job.

The beer project went well, and we had Glen's cellar about half full of bottled potatoes. Every once in a while one of the bottles would pop its cap, sure evidence that the fermentation process was working. We were satisfied with the product. We were not satisfied with our partner, Glen, because he managed to drink it nearly as fast as it was bottled. We told him to save us some—after all, it was our potato money. He finally agreed. We also agreed to operate on the cat, come the next Saturday night.

About a week before the beer manufacturing pact, Mary Helen pulled a big surprise and told me that she thought she was pregnant. Happy days! She would be about two months along and decided to get a doctor appointment as soon as she could. One Saturday morning, she said she didn't feel well. I suggested the doctor. She said, "No, I'll wait."

Glen and Gay came over and Glen brought a dozen bottles of our home brew, Gay fixed a pork heart and Donna had the shrimp soaking in vinegar. The party was set. We started early and Mary Helen started with us. Excusing herself she said she was going upstairs to lie down. I asked her again about the doctor. Again she said no. We thought it might be morning sickness, but this was in the evening. We all assured ourselves that it was nothing serious.

After the twelve beers were gone, Glen suggested we go get some more so we went across the street to help him carry it back. When we got there, the old tom cat was locked up on the Fuller's back porch. Full of home brew, and by now brave as could be, we decided it was time for surgery. Glen found a pillow case and we managed to get the squalling, scratching cat in the bag. A sack full of beer in one hand and the cat in the other we took off for our private operating room— Bechdolt's kitchen table.

I went upstairs, reeking of beer, and checked up on my wife. She told me to go away. Said she thought she was having a miscarriage. I turned away and again asked about the doctor. She said, ". . . maybe, check with me after while." I left and went down stairs. Bill, in the meantime, got out his surgery kit and sterilized the instruments in some water and disinfectant. I had managed to get some pentobarbitol sodium from the pharmacy at school, and with a syringe from our kit we gave the tom cat a shot to put him to sleep. I heard Mary Helen moan through the hole in the dining room ceiling. I gulped down the rest of my beer and ran upstairs in a hurry. She said for me to call the doctor; she was awfully sick. I called; the doctor was not in but I was assured that he would come to the house as soon as he could—maybe in an hour. Mary Helen told me to go away. I did and I went back down stairs. Bill was ready, and the cat appeared to be in a deep sleep.

Now, besides being neophite surgeons, we thought we were also qualified anesthetists. We drank another bottle of beer, and we tossed a coin to see who would make the initial incision. Bill won. He made a big bold incision just like the book described. The cat let out a scream you could have heard a block away. Our expertise in anesthesia was at an all time low! At the same time the cat squalled, he sprayed urine all over the kitchen. Like a cloud of fog, that awful odor of cat urine filtered up through the hole in the ceiling to where my poor wife was suffering. We caught the cat and wrapped him in a towel and now it was my turn to cut. I made my move and while Bill forcibly held down the half asleep tom cat, I finished the job and removed both testicles. We were successful. We drank one more beer which we sure didn't need. We put the cat back in the sack and Glen carried him home and put him back on his screened in porch. Gay went with me upstairs to check on Mary Helen. The whole house smelled like pick-led hearts and potato beer, neatly blended with the horrible odor of cat urine. Gay left saying if I needed her to yell and she would come right away. As she walked down the porch steps, a car pulled up in front of the house. It was the doctor.

The doctor stepped inside the door. He gasped at the odor and looked quizingly at me for an answer. I told him I was sorry about the bad smell but a frightened cat had sprayed in the kitchen. I didn't tell him why or how come. He tended my poor sick wife, gave her an injection, confirmed she was miscarrying and left orders for her care. She soon went to sleep, and I went down and helped Bill clean up the mess. Donna was mad. She didn't speak to either of us for two days. She went upstairs to check on Mary Helen. The party was over.

Mary Helen felt better after a day or so, Donna and Gay and M.H. eventually forgave us and things got back to near normal. We didn't see Glen again for a couple of weeks, but when we did he gave us some startling news. It seems that we had castrated the wrong cat. Our patient was a registered cat that belonged to a neighbor. She used him for a breeding stud. We chuckled; his sex days were over. The other old tom continued to carry on his howling, loving and fighting but we decided we had done enough.

Some months after the tom cat surgery episode, and the sad-ness and pain of the miscarriage had passed, Mary Helen told me that she thought she was pregnant again. I told her to get to the doctor as fast as she could to be sure, since she had miscarried, naturally, we wanted everything to be all right. She agreed to make an appoint-ment the next day. That night when we went downstairs to visit with Bill and Donna, Mary Helen told Donna about her suspected condi-tion. Donna laughed, looked at Bill, and said, "There must be some-thing in the water we both drank because I think I'm that way too!"

Bill laughed out loud and he boomed, ". . . must have been one hell of a party, sounds like you both got that way the same night!"

Donna tried to shut him up but he kept kidding both girls and finally said to me, "Jack, let's drink a beer and celebrate."

Donna responded immediately, "What do you have to celebrate? We already have two kids, you know." She asked Mary Helen if she had been to the doctor yet for a pregnancy test. Mary Helen told her she intended making an appointment the next day.

Turning back to the girls, as he reached into the refrigerator for the beer, Bill laughed and said, "I have a great idea that will save us some money." That statement caused us all to listen. He continued, "Why can't we do a rabbit test ourselves? We can use Debby's pet rabbit." Debby was Donna and Bill's little girl. "All we have to do is inject some urine into the rabbit and in so many hours cut her open. If you are pregnant, there will be follicles in the rabbit's ovaries."

Donna jumped at that remark and said, "Bill, you're crazy, that's the kids' pet. If you do anything like that, you are the one to tell them their rabbit's dead."

Almost before Donna was through with her remark, little Debby came running into the room, big tears in her eyes, yelling, "Daddy, please don't hurt my rabbit."

The issue was closed. Debby spent the next day guarding her bunny and both girls went to the doctor. The rabbit got a reprieve; both girls were pregnant. The babies were due, by the doctor's count, late in the summer.

We eventually finished the junior year. We closed the apartment and went home to Portsmouth for the summer. I looked forward to a full time summer job with Dr. Karr. Mary Helen looked forward to having our baby and a rest from college and housekeeping.

Karr was glad I was back and one time I overheard him say to one of his good clients, "By God, Jack Martin is going to be one darned good veterinarian." That statement was more than enough reward to me coming from Owen Karr himself.

Doc, as I called him, had alerted his clients about my coming for the summer. He told them, particularly the farmers, about me and my education up to that point. He asked them if they would accept me as an intern, with the understanding that if I attended one of their sick animals, and did not know what to do for it, I would proceed no farther and call him in on the case. Most agreed to the situation. It was a blessing for both of us. He got some rest; I got some great on-the-job training.

One night during office hours we had a very heavy schedule. After the last person had gone, we still had a cesarean section to do and a cat with a broken leg to splint. Karr had promised the cat's owner he could pick it up in the morning. The last patient walked out the door and as Doc was ready to go to the surgery, the phone rang. The caller was Carl Morton—he had a cow down with milk fever. He said over the phone, " . . . come right away, Doc, she's really bad off . . . ." I would hear the same words hundreds of times later in my career.

Karr thought a moment and finally said, "Jack, take my car and go to Carl's place and treat his cow. If you have any problem at all call me and I'll try to help you out." I was elated.

After getting directions to the farm, and being sure I had the proper medicine for milk fever, I ran out of the office to the car through a downpour of rain. Lightning flashed and thunder pounded like the guns of war. It was a miserable night to be on the roads. Ignoring the elements, I drove off on my first professional call. I was excited, yet a little apprehensive, hoping I would make no mistakes. The closer I got to Morton's place the shakier I got. I thought of a thousand complications before I drove the ten miles through the dark stormy night to the sick cow. Finally I got to the farm, drove into the driveway up to the house and honked the car horn to announce my arrival. We made it a practice to sound the horn rather than getting out because not all farm dogs were friendly. I got no response. I blew the horn again, this time longer. Still no answer. I knew they were expecting me and through the drawn window shades in the front room I could see light. Finally I got out of the car and ran through the rain to the front porch and knocked on the door. Still no response. I knocked once more and as I did, a bolt of lightning flashed and in the brilliance of the storm's light, I was confronted by a person standing not two feet from me staring me right in the face. My God I was scared! Cold sweat broke out on my hands and face and more or less in self defense, I forced a very weak, "Hello."

At that same instant, as the lightning flashed and the thunder boomed, Mr. Morton opened the shade drawn door and flooded the porch with light. Obviously glad that I was there to treat his sick cow, he said, "Hi, Doc, wait 'till I get a flashlight and we'll go to the barn." Still shaking and alarmed I suddenly realized that the figure standing by me on the porch, now bathed in light from the open door, was a life-sized statue of the Virgin Mary. The Mortons were devout Catholics!

I gathered my composure, treated the cow, collected Karr's money and drove back to the office. Doc was just finishing the c-section when I walked in and he asked me about my call. Before I could make any comments, he said, "I didn't figure you would have any complications or run up against anything unusual—that cow gets milk fever every time she comes fresh."

I thought about his remarks for just a moment and then said, "Nope, just a routine case." It had been a grand summer and with Karr's tutoring, I learned a lot.

On August fourteenth Mary Helen went into labor. I took her to the hospital and told her I would be back as soon as I delivered a calf at the Rapp dairy farm.

I delivered a fine big Holstein heifer calf, and by the time I got back to the hospital, Mary Helen's doctor delivered us a beautiful baby girl. We named her Teresa Lynn.

Now, none of these happenings had anything to do with the circus and up until now, the circus aspect of veterinary medicine had never entered my mind. That would all change, and our lives would change too.

MY INTRODUCTION TO THE CIRCUS

We went back to college—the DVM degree just a year away. One morning just before leaving for my classes, Mary Helen asked me an unusual question. "Do you like the circus?"

"Of course I do—everybody likes a circus." The subject had never come up before and puzzled, I asked her, "How come you ask such a question?" Unknowingly, this conversation was to play a major role in our lives.

Excited by my answer, she beamed, "That's great! Let's make a deal! I'll go to the horse shows with you if you go to the circus with me." I felt that was a good arrangement, since she seemed to know more about circuses than I did. At the same time it crossed my mind the circuses had animals and somebody had to doctor them too.

Without waiting for me to utter another word, she said, "I have a girlfriend that is a circus star." This was the first I had ever heard of this and then she told me about her friend.

"One summer, when I was about seven years old, the Cole Brothers Circus came to Portsmouth. The big circus train that came to town during the night was parked on a side track next to a public park, only a block from my house. My Uncle Henri and I sat on my front porch watching the excitement and commotion of this monstrous organization. It was like we had ring-side seats! Animals were everywhere, expertly tended to by their handlers. There were a lot of horses and ponies, a herd of elephants, camels and donkeys.

"Waiting patiently in the shade of a big oak tree in the park was a man holding two llamas. A group of men carefully unloaded a string of canvas covered wagons and from the roars and growls that came from these darkened dens, it was obvious these were the cages that housed exotic jungle cats.

"In what seemed like utter confusion, mobs of people were moving boxes, loading wagons and getting ready to move the show from the rail siding to the circus lot." Mary Helen paused as if to let the picture of this great spectacle settle in my mind. She looked away— the entire scene seemed to be coming back to her. Then, after a moment, she continued her story. "While Uncle Henri and I were watching all of this, a man and a young girl about my age got off of the train and walked down the street away from the crowd.

"They stopped in front of my house. The man, addressing my uncle, said, 'Sir, we are looking for a dry goods store. I want to buy some yarn. Can you tell us where to go?

"I was absolutely fascinated by these circus people and Uncle Henri and I took them down the street to Marting's department store."

Mary Helen then went on to tell me that meeting these two was the beginning of a lifelong friendship. The man was Ernest Clarke. He was the greatest flying trapeze artist of his time—and, perhaps even of all times! He had the reputation of being one of the first "flyers" to complete the triple somersault from the flying trapeze. His daughter's name was Ernestine, who, in time, made her own reputation as a bareback rider and an aerialist like her daddy.

"Ernestine—or Ernie as she was called—and I developed a friendship that has blossomed, and to this very day, we still write and keep in touch." This conversation brought back vivid memories of the day when I watched them pour the iodine on the tiger's cuts on the Hagenbeck-Wallace Circus. I told her that story and casually mentioned that it would certainly be a challenge to be a circus veterinarian. This had been an interesting conversation, but I soon put it out of my mind. We had other priorities—first, and foremost, finishing our college education. One evening after I got home from school, Mary Helen handed me *The Columbus Dispatch* newspaper. It carried big, blaring full page ads advertising the Ringling Bros. and Barnum & Bailey Circus was coming to Columbus. "Promise me," she said,

"Don't make any plans for that day" as she insisted that we go to the circus and meet her friend Ernestine, who was now advertised as a star performer on that show. We rode the streetcar to the show grounds, and stared with amazement at the vast city of canvas, wagons and fascinating people that were with the show.

It was a world different from anything I had ever seen. Taking my hand, my wife guided me past the front part of the circus, to what she knowingly called the "back yard." Obviously, she knew her way around, and after finding someone who spoke English in that international city of performers and working men, we were directed to the Clarke dressing tent. We met Mrs. Clarke, and she told us Ernestine was a guest of a sorority for the day and wouldn't be back until time for the afternoon show. Ernie's mother remembered Mary Helen and suggested we stay for the show and visit with them later in the day. Regretfully, we could not stay, as I had to be in classes that afternoon. And for that matter, we were so poor we didn't have enough money to buy a ticket to the circus! That day, the circus captured my attention as nothing I had ever done before. We wandered around the lot and looked at the long line of elephants, wagons painted red with the show's logo, "The Greatest Show On Earth," painted on each one, camels, acres of canvas, with breeze-blown flags topping each center pole, zebras, ponies and many other animals. In a tent by themselves were cage after cage of lions and tigers, all rumbling to themselves, in talk known only to their kind. A working man cautioned us not to go into that tent, as it was not a safe place for a stranger to be. We heeded his advice and walked over to another tent full of the finest horses I had ever seen. These sleek and fat animals, of several different breeds, were absolutely fascinating to me—a student of their discomforts. Added to this fascinating world were scores of noisy laughing people, young and not so young, playing soccer in the back yard. The confusion of foreign tongues and the sounds from the animals made the entire atmosphere a land of enchantment. Little did I know someday some of these animals would be my patients and many of these people and their families would become lifelong friends. We often talked about that day, and later, after I graduated from college, Mary Helen bought me a book titled, *Circus Doctor*. It was written by Dr. J.Y. Henderson, Chief Veterinarian for Ringling Bros. and Barnum & Bailey Circus. This book soon earned priority space in my desktop book case.

A SAMPLE OF SAWDUST

In the early fifties, my practice covered a large geographical area that included parts of southern Ohio, a large section of western West Virginia and nearly all of eastern Kentucky! As a matter of fact, I was the only college graduated, licensed veterinarian in the Kentucky hill country that did farm animal work. Travel alone over this vast area consumed most of the time. The thought went through my mind if the farmers could bring their animals to me, instead of my going to them, everybody would benefit. In 1953 this idea became reality and I built a new veterinary clinic complex designed to house both small animals and large animals. This idea worked. The client saved money and his or her animals received far better care and treatment at the new facility. I saved time and miles of driving, allowing me to have a little time for recreation.

In due time I bought a horse, then another one and soon I had several good American Saddle Horses. I employed a trainer, and the Martin Veterinary Clinic Stable became well known. We spent most weekends on the horse show circuit.

We also pursued other escapes besides the horse shows to relieve the tension of long hours and hard work. True to my word to Mary Helen, we went to every circus that came close to us. We were fortunate that Jim Hetzer, owner of a circus and a theatrical booking agency in Huntington, West Virginia, had the contract each year to supply acts for Ashland Oil Company's Christmas show. These acts were the best in the land. Big name performers vied for contracts for this Christmas date and, through our friend Hetzer, we soon became friends with many of them. Included on this list of notables were such famous circus names as the George Hannefords and the Stephensons. Stephensons had, besides their riding act, the top dog act of the times. Bucky Steele was a repeater there, with his bears. Gee Gee Engesser Powell, and her Husky Dogs, Ferry Forst, the illusionist, along with his lovely daughters and wife were part of the group. Kaiche Namba, a tiny Japanese gentleman, was a head balancer and soon became one of our closest friends. These acts all came from different shows, and before long, Mary Helen and I were pretty well versed on who was who and with what show. We met many that were not in the animal business. This list included the world famous clowns Otto Griebling and Lou Jacobs. Otto was, beyond a doubt, one of the funniest men I have ever known, whether he was doing his show routine or being just plain Otto as my house guest in later years. Lou Jacobs, who owned probably the best known clown face in the world, was one of the nicest, kindest men I have ever known. He too spread laughs and joy to many with his famous comedy routines. He also was a guest in our home. Through other channels, we met such stars as the Aerial Hustries—a high act with a sway pole routine that was superb. The Alcedos were another high act and featured Wilfred Alcedo, Rusty Johnson and Jimmy Lloyd. Later Jimmy Lloyd, who lived with us one winter, left to join the Terrel Jacobs Circus out of Indiana. About mid-season, he left that show and went over to the Hagen Brothers Circus for the rest of the summer. Before Hagen's tour was over, Jimmy was killed by an elephant on that show—making us realize that not all circus life was glitz and glitter! Rusty is still our friend. The list of friends grew larger and one day Rose Alexander, of the Flying Alexanders, mentioned to Virginia Hustrie that the Martins knew more people in the circus world than most of the agents and promoters did.

After some of those dates we invited many of the performers to visit our house for a party after the show was over, and most of them did come. Our guest book reads like a Who's Who of sawdust and spangles.

It was but a matter of time until some of the animal acts had need for a veterinarian. Jim Hetzer, without a moment's hesitation, strongly recommended me. I treated Kirby's chimps for colds, Steele's bears for bad teeth and Stephenson's dogs for periodic veterinary needs. It was not uncommon for the phone to ring, necessitating that I would conduct a veterinary consultation with some circus animal owner over the phone.

As our association with these circus people went on, still enthralled by Dr. Henderson's book, I pursued the circus animal business and it wasn't long until I was doing a lot of that work right at my own place. The concept of my clinic appealed to the show people, and they soon realized they could bring any animal—large or small, exotic or domestic—to me for treatment. They also found out they had room to park their trailers and trucks on my clinic property, while I was attending to their needs. After visiting one of these shows, and transposed back into the real world, I read and reread every page of Dr. Henderson's book. I tried to imagine what I would do if I was ever faced with a major kind of circus veterinary challenge. "Doc," as the book said his colleagues called him, was indeed—in my mind—the most fascinating veterinarian in the world. I was determined to meet Dr. Henderson and perhaps even follow in his footsteps as a circus doctor.

"HEY DOC, THERE'S ANOTHER DOC OUT HERE TO SEE YOU"

The Ringling Bros. and Barnum & Bailey Circus fell on hard times in the late fifties. However, by the grace of some determined souls, and a few monetary benefactors, it was back on the road after labor strikes closed the show in Pittsburgh. This time, instead of traveling by rail, the show traveled by trucks. Quite a letdown for The Greatest Show On Earth. Early one cold spring, the Ringling circus advertised they would show in Huntington, West Virginia—just fifteen miles from home. This time we had the money for tickets, and we went early to see the show. Mary Helen's friend Ernie was no longer with this circus, and the only other person I had a personal interest in was Dr. Henderson.

Looking for help, one of the first people I saw was one of the "little people"—an endearing circus term for midgets or dwarfs. We introduced ourselves to him and asked him where I could find their veterinarian. I also asked him his name. Shaking hands with us both, he replied, "Around here they call me Slippery Socks." He took us in tow, and cheerfully led us to the backyard. Making our way through the clutter of trailers, wagons, and what seemed to us utter confusion, he pointed to a red trailer and said, "That's where Doc lives." When he got to the trailer he yelled, "Hey, Doc, there is another Doc out here to see you." I knocked on the door and we were greeted by a beautiful, red haired Mrs. Henderson. She called her husband, we were invited inside and that's how we met J.Y. and Martha. The year was 1959, and this was the beginning of a lifelong friendship, not only with the circus doctor himself, but his entire family. They became part of our lives and our family and we became part of theirs.

The doctor insisted we call him "J.Y." He said that was his name and that the initials stood for nothing—his daddy liked the sound of the two initials, when he was born, and he had been J.Y. ever since. J.Y. was a Texan and, most of all, he was a horseman. I related my past experience and told him that the reason that I had become a veterinarian was because of my fascination with the horse. This mutual love for the horse forever sealed our friendship. He sized me up and told me to call him "J.Y." However, most of the show people called him "Doc." The name, "Doc Henderson," was legend in the circus world. He later tagged me with a nickname, "Jackson." We had a nice visit with his wife, Martha, and after a while Dr. Henderson took Mary Helen and me in hand and gave us a tour of what the circus people called their back yard.

Then it was show time and when Harold Ronk, the famous, very talented singing ringmaster, announced, "Children of all ages, John Ringling North presents Ringling Bros. and Barnum & Bailey Circus—The Greatest Show On Earth," the magic and the intrigue captured me. Mary Helen and I were enchanted as, one by one, the procession of performers paraded past us as we sat in choice seats that J.Y. provided. I was really in love with this business.

After the performance was over, J.Y. introduced us to many of the performers and show personnel. Trevor Bale—a really nice gentleman—was the lion and tiger trainer. His reputation, we later learned, as an animal trainer, was legend. "Deacon" Blanchfield, a very religious man and hence his name, was another of J.Y.'s good friends. Deacon had been the train master when the show moved on rails, and was probably one of the most experienced circus men on the show. Later, he retired to the Circus World Museum in Baraboo, Wisconsin, where he demonstrated his talent, loading and unloading horsedrawn circus wagons on the train. Blanchfield was soon to become one of my very good friends too. Other stars we met included Mr. Unus, the man who balanced himself on one finger; Charlie Moroski, perhaps the best horse trainer in the world, his wife Gina, and Harold "Tuffy" Genders, an ex-flying trapeze artist, now general manager of the circus. We renewed our friendship with Dean MacMurray, formerly with Mills Brothers Circus, now the office manager for Ringling. Besides our friends Otto Greibling and Lou Jacobs, we became friends with Prince Paul, Paul Jung, Frankie Saluto, Freddie Freeman, Danny Chapman and Mark Anthony—all in clown alley. Many others were to become our friends over the years.

Splashed with the glitter of the circus and fascinated by the people we had just met, we said our good-byes and drove back to Ashland—and reality. On the way home I admitted to my wife that I was envious of our newfound friend, Dr. Henderson, and his job. Later that night, trying to go to sleep, I couldn't get the brassy music of the circus band director, Merle Evans, out of my mind. The magic would not go away.

The Ringling show was the crown jewel of circuses—this was the glitter bunch. I had yet to experience the mud show, or the smaller traveling tented circus that crisscrossed our country every day—entertaining people, trying to pay its way. Most of these smaller shows played a different town every day, rain or shine. The performers and working men on these outfits put in long hard hours, driving overland at night—catching a few hours sleep when they could. Then it was another day, setting the show up and playing the town. Long hours later, the last show ended and the glamour of the circus was gone. Everyone, performers, as well as working men, went to work tearing it down, loading it up and moving the circus to the next town. It was a hard life, appreciated only by those that did it.

The animals had hard times too with this constant moving, but they soon acclimated to it and really did better on the road than in winter quarters! In their support I must say, right here, that circus animals are probably the best cared for and best treated animals in the world. Generally speaking, no expense is ever spared when it comes to their care. My exposure to this kind of circus was yet to come.

MILLS BROTHERS CIRCUS

As we got more and more involved with the circus, Mary Helen and I joined an organization called the Circus Fans Association. The CFA is made up of just what it says—circus fans whose one and only interest is to live, breath and eat circus! The CFA climaxes each year with a convention where the members exhibit circus collectibles, photographs of shows—past and present—and swap tales or gossip or as they say in the business, "Cut up jackpots." A different circus usually entertains the convention each year. In 1959 the meeting was to be held in Clarksburg, West Virginia. The hosting show was to be the Mills Brothers Circus, currently out of Jefferson, Ohio. Clarksburg isn't far from Ashland, so we made a hotel reservation, sent in our convention registration fees, and headed for a weekend of entertainment that would forever change a part of our lives.

The Mills Brothers Circus was a large tented circus owned by three brothers—Jack, Jake and Harry Mills. It traveled overland by trucks and was one of those shows that everyone in the business affectionately called a mud show. Jack ran the circus, Jake was in charge of some of the management and productions and brother Harry Mills had the concessions. Howdy Earhart was the promoter who set the dates and locations. Wilson Storey, a retired animal trainer, was the general agent and he, with his extensive circus back ground, along with Jack Mills, did most of the talent hiring. This experienced staff and the superb collection of yearly imported European acts, made this circus outstanding.

The show lot in Clarksburg was downtown along the river, and as we approached it from the town's main street, we drove down a steep road. Below us we could see the entire layout of sparkling white tents, trucks and trailers nestled at the foot of the hill. Behind the tents, along the riverbank in the shade of some trees, a herd of elephants was staked out on a picket line. I stopped the car for a moment and we watched these huge animals weaving back and forth, rumbling their contentment while they ate their hay.

We drove down the steep grade, parked our car and mingled with the crowd. Members of the Circus Fans Association wore name tags and, of course, it wasn't long before we were all calling each other by our first names. Most of these people had attended several conventions in previous years. They knew a lot of the performers and, with their help, we met about everyone connected with the show, including the Mills brothers themselves.

The actual program was excellent, but not nearly as fascinating to us as was the maze of ropes and canvas, the trucks and tons of equipment. We watched the general hustle of the workers. It seemed to us like well organized, utter confusion. But the show people captivated us the most.

For beginners, the elephant superintendent was Captain Virgil Seagraves—home town, Ashland, Kentucky! Immediately, we became friends. His helper was Lou Turner and he too took us under his wing.

We met an older performer named Herman Joseph. Herman was a famous clown, and in makeup he dressed like a hobo, in baggy rags and a tattered hat. His show experience dated back through several old circuses including the Barnum & Bailey Circus —forerunner of today's Ringling Bros. and Barnum & Bailey show. Most of his entire life, beginning when he was a very young man, had been spent in the circus. He was a very quiet man and seemed to be searching for a friend. He found one in Mary Helen and stayed in touch with her until he died some years later. One of his best gags came during the grand parade—or in circus lingo the Spec—as it moved around the hippodrome track. Mr. Joseph was the last man in the grand parade. He trudged along just behind the elephants appearing to have a job to do. In one hand he carried a huge scoop shovel, appearing ready to pick up any of the gigantic droppings as the big animals paraded their way before the audience. He kept his other hand busy, under his nose, whisking away the imaginary odor that was sure to follow these big brutes! It was always good for a laugh. Herman Joseph trouped with Mills until they closed the show. He was really a great clown and never received a lot of credit as such until later years when his talent was recognized.

And then we met CoCo. He was much younger than Herman Joseph and talked with a heavy British accent. CoCo was a third generation clown born in Rega, Latvia. His father, and his father before him, were well known performers in England and on the continent. CoCo had a partner named Victor Lewis. Victor was the brother of Harry Mills' wife, June. He teamed with CoCo as part of the clown routine. Like most of the performers, Victor had another job on the show. He sold concessions and drove the canvas truck on overland trips. Both of these people were later to become involved in my family's personal lives.

Other people whom we met that day included John Zerbini and his family, from France. John was the lion trainer and his entire wardrobe, when he presented his act, was a small leopard skin loincloth. He showed under the name of Tarzan—certainly fitting for such an act. Later on Tarzan was very successful and owned a large circus of his own.

Other new acquaintances included some show girls that CoCo had gathered for Mills while visiting in England. Rita was one of these girls; she eventually married the elephant trainer Virgil Seagraves. Another, Christine, married Paul Hudson, who was the boss canvas man and who operated the pony ride. CoCo also brought his step daughter Julia from England with him. Once here in America she met and married Mauricio Drougett, a world class juggler from South America. Other new acquaintances were Pedro and Gherta, an aerial act from Germany and Beppe and Paulo, who were "kinkers" or contortionists. They were also of German origin. Rudy Dockey was an

Austrian, who had boxer dogs who played basketball. Paul Nelson, who was superintendent of horses, was, like me, a Kentuckian. He handled all of the horse acts. Bill McCullough worked for Harry Mills in concessions and was a truck driver when the show moved. We also met George Strongman, who handled the front office affairs and, of course, the Mills brothers. This made up quite an interesting contingent of people.

Before the day was over, Rudy Dockey came to see me with a health problem with his dogs. His prolific Sissy was about to have another litter of puppies. This was his continuing source of replacement dog performers. Sissy was a hard worker and when she was not pregnant, worked in the act. Her one reward, for all her strain, was that she got to live in the tiny trailer with her boss Rudy. I examined the dog and finally prescribed a vitamin supplement and suggested she be allowed to rest longer between litters and be given a cleaner place to live. Dockey agreed with my suggestion for better hygiene and responded in a heavy German accent, since I was now Sissy's personal doctor, he would move some of his beer out of the way and make her a new bed. I was pleased—Sissy was one of my very first circus patients.

The elephant man, Seagraves, came to me a little while later and we had some elephant talk. I didn't tell him I was not too knowledgeable about "bulls," the circus term for either sex of elephants—I didn't discourage him either. He called me "Doc" and, now that we were on a first name basis, I called him "K.Y." K.Y. said that one of his charges, India, was prone to have chills and that very day she was sick. Could I help him? Now, right there, if I was going to be a circus doctor, I had to come up with some fast answers. I pondered a very short time and remembered a book I had read written by an elephant handler in the teak woods of Burma. In his book he mentioned any time one of his animals got sick, he would give it a pint of gin! Well I knew from my war experiences in Burma, the only reason we Americans thought the British drank gin was because they couldn't get good whiskey! This thought in mind, I told Captain Seagraves to get a pint of whiskey and give India about one half of the bottle. I assured him the treatment would work and she would be OK. Later, between shows, an inebriated elephant trainer showed up and told me his sick India was just fine but he thought that a half pint was too much for her, so he cut the dose to 4 ounces and then proceeded to drink the rest himself! An unorthodox treatment at the best, but on the spur of the moment that was all I knew to tell him. My first elephant case was a success. Captain Seagraves eventually recovered too.

Later that evening, just before the night show, Mary Helen and I were visiting with Chris and Paul Hudson. They were at the pony ride concession and were busy giving rides to the little kids. While the ponies were going around the ring with their paying guests, Jack Mills came up and thanked me for attending to his ailing elephant. Jack's dark whiskers made him appear to be unshaven. He unbuttoned his shirt collar and loosened his neck tie as he hunched up in his coat to cover the chill of the cool mountain air. He certainly didn't look the part of the circus owner, but it was a typical picture of Jack Mills. After he had thanked me for helping him, he said, "It's a good convention—ain't it?" He was certainly not aware of my medication. I had been warned that he condoned no drinking on his show. He asked about my fee and I promptly told him what I had done was my small token for the joys that Mary Helen and I had that day with his people and his show. Jack Mills liked a dollar, knew how to make one and knew how to keep it after he got it. He was a frugal man. My free services were really appreciated. During our conversation he asked about my past, my circus experience and my intentions. I told him the straight truth and that I was enjoying a struggling mixed practice in northern Kentucky and aspired to someday be a veterinarian who did circus animal medicine. He hesitated and then told me that on occasion he needed a veterinarian, especially for the horses and ponies. I asked myself, why particularly the ponies, when he owned all of these other exotic animals like elephants and chimpanzees? He added, before I could say much, "You know, doctor, the money from this pony ride moves my show!" He meant, of course, that the ride was so lucrative that it paid for the gasoline for all of the trucks and vehicles! Looking back on this, years later, and then far wiser about the circus business, I could appreciate this because the quickest way to a little kid's heart was with a pony. Case in point, look what the first ride did to me! Jack Mills finished his conversation with me by adding, "Doctor, you and your wife feel free to be guests here any time you want to. You and Mrs. Martin are always welcome on my show." Jack Mills was a nice man and was always ready to greet us when we came to visit.

After the night performance was over, we watched the men take the show down, roll up the Big Top and other tents, load them, the props and the animals into the trucks and start on the long night drive over the West Virginia mountains to the next town. The steep grade up from the river bank to the main Clarksburg street proved no problem for the heavy overloaded trucks. Virgil Seagraves, with his elephants, were standing by, ready with a head shove when a truck faltered leaving the lot. Finally only the generator truck and the bull truck were left. Then the generator was shut down and the lot was in total darkness. After that truck made it up the hill, K.Y. loaded his bulls with the aid of a flashlight and drove away. The magic was gone. Mary Helen and I said our good-byes and drove back to Kentucky and the reality of my kind of veterinary medicine, never realizing this trip would, in time, lead to many circus adventures.

Later on in the season, the Mills Brothers Circus played in several towns close to us and we visited the show at every opportunity. Jack Mills could depend on me and I did some minor veterinary jobs for him.

Toward the end of the season, the circus was in Zanesville, Ohio, playing its way back toward their winter quarters in Jefferson, north on the shores of Lake Erie. Jack talked to me and suggested we come to the opening at Easter time. He said he had a new baby elephant on order and we both needed the newspaper publicity—he for his circus, me for my budding circus practice. We assured him we would be there.

By this time, we had many friends on Mills and suggested to CoCo and his friends, Victor Lewis and George Strongman, that they stop for a visit, after the circus closed and they were on their way south to Florida for the winter.

Fall turned to winter and the snows came. I forgot about circuses and went about my daily work delivering calves, spaying cats and dogs, fixing broken legs and giving vaccinations. Nothing was routine—all of it, even after eight or nine years, was still exciting.

Close to the end of March, Jack Mills called me and reminded me that his show began its new season during Easter weekend. He hoped we still planned to be there for the opening. I assured him, we intended to be there and thanked him for remembering us.

On the Wednesday before Easter, Mary Helen and I drove north to Jefferson. The north winds over Lake Erie blew bitter cold and the last of the winter's snow squalls were in the air. It didn't seem to be circus weather to me.

Most of our Mills friends were there, and the opening show was set for Saturday. To Jack Mills' delight, the baby elephant was the subject of a feature article in the *Cleveland Plain Dealer* newspaper, wonderful free publicity! The article, which incidentally included my name, made a big issue that Mills Brothers Circus owners, all Cleveland natives, had taken delivery of the new baby elephant at the Cleveland airport on the previous Monday.

K.Y. Seagraves told me about the baby's arrival. According to him, it was a bitter cold, wind swept day when the plane arrived. The baby was taken off of the airplane and paraded back and forth for the press and visitors to see. The entire Mills family was there, including Jack's daughter and her friends, and every one wanted to do something for the new arrival. They fed it popcorn and peanuts and candy bars. Certainly not the best diet for a baby elephant. After all of the hoopla of the press, the baby bull—called a "punk" in circus language— was loaded into K.Y.'s truck and driven to winter quarters.

Winter quarters was a county fair grounds and the elephants, Burma, India, Jenny, Lena and Roxi, were housed in one of the old cattle barns. This barn was drafty and the only heat came from a portable gas space heater set along the wall in front of the animals. To help keep the drafts and cold air out of the building, old hay and manure was heaped behind the bulls and along the wall directly in front of them. The little elephant was unloaded and introduced to the herd. Burma, K.Y.'s favorite, soon adopted the baby and it was decided to chain the new arrival between her and Jenny on the picket line. The five giants, loaded with curiosity and affection, gently examined the new arrival with their trunks. The Mills brothers were ecstatic; they had a new featured attraction, a lot of good press and a new season ready to start.

The baby settled in Monday night and after a light feed seemed content. Tuesday morning brought more cold, snow flurries and wind. Most of the chill was taken out of the bull barn by the manure pile insulation and the gas heater. Herds of mice ran up and down in the old bedding and maybe made friends with the elephants—surely contrary to the belief that mice and pachyderms don't mix! The baby didn't eat too well and K.Y. suggested to Jack Mills that, "Maybe Doc Martin ought to look at her as soon as he gets in town."

Late Wednesday evening, Mary Helen and I pulled into the fairgrounds, and we had no sooner passed through the main gate, when we were met by Jack and Jake Mills and Virgil Seagraves. They told me about their new baby and said that they were concerned that it didn't seem to feel well. I went straight to the elephant barn.

The baby was perhaps three feet tall at her shoulders. Her tiny little trunk wasn't much larger than a garden hose and her dark eyes were as big as dinner cups. She was visibly sick and obviously in a lot of pain, with what I assumed were abdominal cramps. The pain would hit her and she would groan and cry out—elephant tears rolled down her little cheeks. It hurt me to see such suffering. I made my initial examination and told an anxious Jack Mills that she had pneumonia and some sort of an intestinal disturbance—I added that the baby elephant was critically sick and my prognosis was guarded.

I did what I could to ease the pain. I covered the baby with blankets and administered antibiotics for the pneumonia. Imagining the little animal to be like a human baby with the colic, I gave her an antispasmodic, to ease her cramps. When the medicine did its work, she relaxed and temporarily stopped the awful crying and suffering. The baby elephant died late that night, in a dark cold drafty barn, far away from her native tropical land of India. K.Y. and I both were emotionally upset. Jack Mills' only comment was, "That's a lot of money to lay there dead—ain't it?"

The next morning I suggested to Jack that we do an autopsy, in case the insurance company needed some facts. He thought this was a good idea and, after dragging the body out behind the big barn, I went to work. Postmortem examination revealed pneumonia in both lungs. This still didn't account for the colic-like symptoms that caused my patient so much pain, so I opened up her stomach and small intestine. The stomach was full of candy bar wrappers and pop bottle tops. The upper part of the small intestine contained more of the same plus an impaction of what appeared to be peanut shells. This baby had died because somebody thought they were being good to her. I made a full report to Jack Mills. The case was closed. The show opened on Saturday and a new season was under way. The baby elephant was never mentioned again.

Mary Helen and I continued following the Mills Circus whenever they were in our neighborhood. They had a good season, playing their normal route through Indiana, Ohio, Pennsylvania, New Jersey, New York and a few dates in West Virginia. They showed six days a week—never on Sunday—and always did a good business.

It was 1960 and the season closed. Mary Helen and I again invited CoCo and Victor Lewis to stop by on their way to Florida for the winter. They came, intending to stay for the weekend and stayed six months! The two clowns were quite an attraction in our town and a newspaper story about them made quite a play about our daughter Terri having two professional clowns for her baby sitters.

Bill McCullough was killed by another truck when he was trying to repair his circus truck on the New Jersey Turnpike. Victor left and moved to Sarasota, married a nice girl and eventually became a lock-smith. Mary Helen and I introduced CoCo to our friend, Hazel Fannin, here in Kentucky. They married and raised a family and still live here as my neighbors. CoCo went on to become a center ring star on the Greatest Show on Earth, the Ringling Bros. and Barnum & Bailey Circus.

The Mills Brothers Circus finally took down its big top for the last time. Jack and Jake Mills died—Harry is a free lance concessionaire—still in the circus business. I liked the Mills brothers, who in their own way became very good friends of ours. Certainly my experiences with them was part of the foundation for my career in the exotic animal business and the circus.

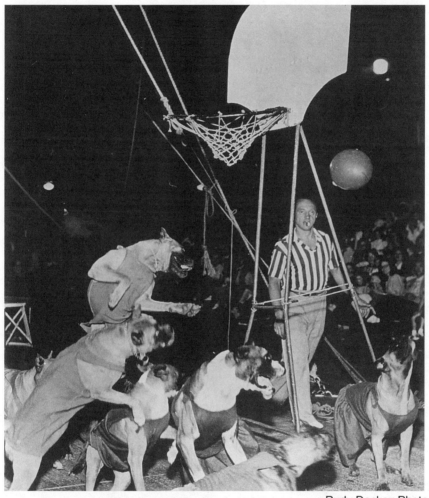

Rudy Dockey and his basketball-playing dogs. Rudy Dockey was the first circus client I worked for and was one of the best dog trainers I ever knew.

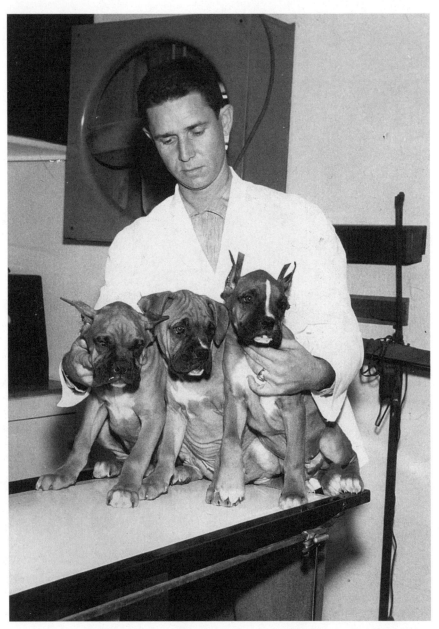

Dr. Martin and three boxer puppies belonging to Rudy Dockey at the Martin Veterinary Clinic. Puppies were shipped there for ear cropping.

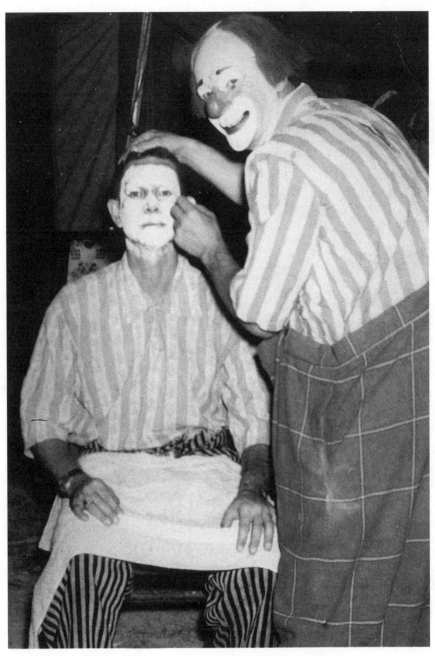

CoCo the clown makes up Dr. Martin for the Spec on the Mills Brothers Circus, 1959.

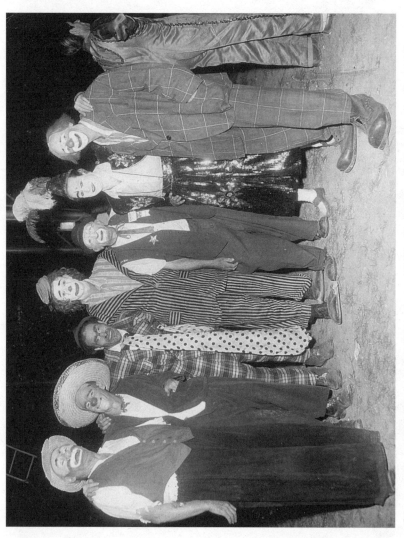

Clown alley, Mills Brothers Circus ca. 1959. (l-r) Harry Baker, two Spanish clowns, Dr. Martin, Herman Joseph, Spanish clown and Coco.

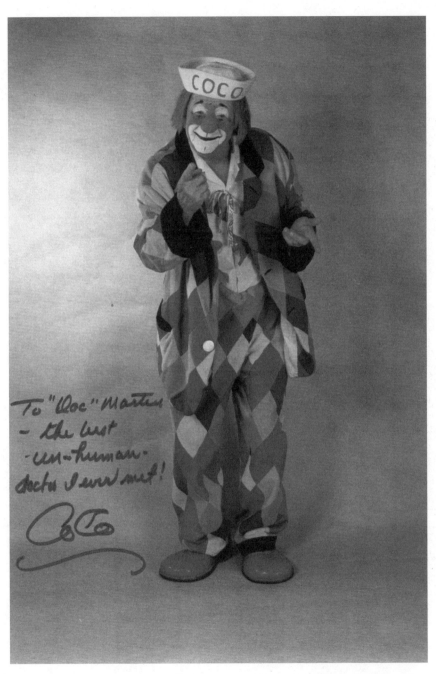

To "Doc" Martin
– the best
– un-human -
doctor I ever met!

CoCo

Michelle Polikovs photo

Michael Polikovs, aka CoCo The Clown, ca. 1995.

MY VERY FIRST JOB FOR RINGLING BROS. CIRCUS

L ate in the fall of 1960, after the Mills Brothers Circus closed for the season, my friend CoCo and I drove to Sarasota. He wanted to visit his stepdaughter and friends and to look for a job. He hoped someway he could get on the Ringling circus. Of course, while we were there, we visited the old Ringling winter quarters, which was in the process of being torn down after the show moved to their new home in Venice. Bulldozers pushed over buildings and heaped the remains in piles, then what was left of that part of circus history was torched! Rotting railroad cars sitting on a siding were nearly hidden by the tall weeds that were growing between the ties and the rusted tracks. Parts of these cars were salvaged and what was left went up in smoke. Old circus wagons—their gilt and paint faded by the hot Florida sun—sunburst wagon wheels by the dozens and props, used in shows past, all came under the bulldozer blade and were piled on the fire. It was sad to see these mementos of this part of Americana lost forever. Later, many of the collectors of circus memorabilia shed tears at the wanton destruction of these artifacts.

While we were in Sarasota, CoCo got an interview with Pat Valdo, a former clown with Ringling, and now a staff executive. CoCo, using his past reputation, and leaning on his father's too, convinced Mr. Valdo to give him a contract for the new season. We drove back to Kentucky; CoCo packed his clothes and said good-bye. My weekend-stayed-for-six-month-house guest—was on his way to the Greatest Show On Earth.

CoCo was a success, and soon gained fame as a star performer, even becoming popular enough to have his picture on the front cover of *The Saturday Evening Post*.

When CoCo got to winter quarters, he met Dr. Henderson and told him he had just spent the winter with a veterinarian who was interested in the circus. J.Y. queried, "Who was that?"

"Doc Martin, up in Ashland, Kentucky."

Surprised, Henderson said, "Jackson Martin?" using the nickname he had given me, "He and his wife are friends of my wife Martha and me!" From this conversation, a lasting friendship blossomed between the clown and the circus doctor.

The 1961 edition of the Greatest Show On Earth moved out of the Venice winter quarters and started north for its new season. In early March, the circus train pulled into Charleston, West Virginia, for a two-day stand. Mary Helen and I caught the show, and this time J.Y. was there. As soon as we walked in the front door of the building, Doc and CoCo saw us. J.Y. rushed to meet us, gave Mary Helen a big kiss and calling me by his favorite name, Jackson, he shook my hand and made us at home. Martha, his pretty, red-haired wife, was not with him but he told us she planned to join him when the show got to New York.

In our initial conversation, he asked me if I was still interested in circus animal work and I told him, "I sure was." I informed him that I had been doing some work at a local amusement park zoo as well as some work for Jim Hetzer's circus and through Hetzer, some of the animal acts that played the local oil company's Christmas dates. My conversation finished, I asked him if he had done "anything exciting."

A big smile came on his face and he said, "Let's go to the Animal Top." Mary Helen looked confused at that term and, he quickly explained that in circus language, the word "top" meant a tent. He continued, "I want to show you some real good Texas horses." Leading the way we went around to the back yard and walked into the big tent that housed all of the animals, except the big cats. The lions and the tigers had a separate tent of their own. We walked through the opening in the end of the big tent and there, tied on a picket line on the right side of the tent, their rear ends facing us, were twenty-four fat and sleek, prime horses, all about the same size, and all the same chestnut color. These were registered American Quarter Horses. All were stallions and all were branded on their hips with the Running W—the brand of the King Ranch in Texas. "Jackson," he said, "This is the liberty act I broke this winter in quarters. I handpicked and bought every one of them myself."

On the left hand side of this tent, each chained by one foot to a cable stretched along the floor, were twenty-one elephants, rocking back and forth, swinging their trunks and looking closely at us strangers. J.Y. reached over and caught Mary Helen's hand and gently pulling her away from one huge elephant said, "Don't get too close to that bitch, she'll hurt you." He hesitated just a minute, and looking directly at the elephant, he said, with some disgust in his voice, "Her name is Targa." It was obvious there was no love affair there! Getting back to his discussion about the new horse act he added, "I broke these horses about the same time you and CoCo were in Sarasota—during the time they were doing away with our old winter home. Its too bad that I didn't know you two were there." Continuing his discussion he said, "Charlie Moroski has this act fine-tuned and he and his wife present them in the show. Tell me what you think of them after the afternoon performance." The act lived up to all J.Y. said it would and Charlie Moroski and Gina, both master show people, made the performance outstanding. J.Y. could rightfully be proud. These King Ranch horses made a great act but now, since the show was playing indoor dates and the horses were stabled where everybody could see them, they caused some embarrassing moments when the stallions got their sex hormones going full blast. John Ringling North, Mr. Circus himself, told Dr. Henderson to have all of the stallions gelded except four. He thought in time these four horses might make exceptional gifts for some of his celebrity friends. It was Henderson's intention to geld these horses when the show spent its long stand in Madison Square Garden in New York City.

Later in the year, J.Y. called me and asked if I would take one of the stallions. The remaining four were still causing problems and John Ringling North was ready to find them a home. Mr. North elected to give one to his friend the King of Iraq and was open for suggestions for placing the other three. Without hesitating J.Y. suggested they give one to Mrs. Ferguson, a granddaughter of Andrew Carnegie and the lady whose family owned Cumberland Island just off the coast of northern Florida. It was Mrs. Ferguson's intention to turn her stallion loose among the island's wild horse herd, to upgrade their offspring. And then he told Mr. North that he thought one should go to Dr. and Mrs. Martin, up in Kentucky! The fourth horse was to stay with the show.

That winter, after the circus was back in winter quarters, we took the horse trailer to Florida and picked up our new stud. The horse Mr. North gave us was named Royal—all of these horses had been named after Texas towns—and by chance, he was the featured horse in the *American Quarter Horse Journal* a few months before we got him. Royal stood at stud for several years at our farm, Jomar, and many of his progeny still dot the eastern Kentucky pastures.

The remaining King Ranch stallion stayed with the show and was mainly used as a replacement horse in case something happened to one of the regulars. He got more roguish and harder to manage as time went on. One vice led to another and he developed an old stud horse trick of wanting to bite at anything he saw. He was like a mean dog! They kept a muzzle on him and generally managed his bad habit until one of the grooms had a finger almost bitten off. J.Y. called me and wanted to know if I would come to Dayton, Ohio, and do the surgery on this horse. Before Dr. Henderson hung up the telephone, he added, "Jackson, it's only fair to tell you he's a real mean bastard!"

Of course, I jumped at the chance. This would be my first job for the Ringling Bros. and Barnum & Bailey Circus.

As I drove along the road to my circus house-call, the memories of two other wild, mean horses that I cared for back in the early '50s came back to me. Surely this circus horse couldn't be as bad as they were. Let me tell you about them.

It was late January—the winter of 1953. It was a hard winter, maybe one of the worst one in years. Just after New Year's Day we had downpours of hard rain that turned the unpaved country roads into quagmires of mud. The creeks were out of their banks and our usually friendly eastern Kentucky countryside was cold and wet and seemed to turn against us. It wasn't a very good time of the year. Then came the big freeze and a deep snow. Everything was white. The creeks were freezing over but in a few open places in the ice, you could see the rushing muddy water of the heavy rains making its way toward the Big Sandy and Ohio Rivers. Only the mail carrier, a brave few who worked in town at the refinery or the steel mill and the local farm veterinarian, dared venture out. Most of the refinery workers and the steel mill hands "laid off" due to the weather and stayed at home—as a local saying went, "Close to the fire." I had no choice. My animal patients got sick any time and like the mailman, "through rain or snow, or dark of night" I made my rounds.

One Monday morning, just after the big freeze, I finished treating the sick animals in my office and got ready to make my country rounds. I had two farm calls to make. The first was up on Bear Creek, to examine and treat some sick half grown pigs. The second call was to attend to a cow that just aborted her calf and had to have her afterbirth removed.

As I packed my medical bag with what I thought I would need for the day's work, outside my office I could hear the wind howl as it drove blinding gusts of snow and ice against the building. I looked out the window of my exam room at a thermometer I had put there just a few days earlier and the bitterness of the outside suddenly became more real than ever. The mercury was pegged at fifteen degrees above zero! That was very cold for our country. It was an awful day to be outside but I had to go. Driving on the paved roads would be bad enough, but the graveled ones, which made up most of our rural roads, were even worse.

The gusting, swirling snow flurries made it almost impossible to see as I drove toward my first visit but, with the windshield wipers on the car working at full speed, I pushed on through the snow drifts, skidding and sliding. I was about six miles toward my pig call on the Bear Creek Road when suddenly my car broke through the ice into a deep mud hole under the snow and came to a jolting stop. I was stuck. Disgusted with this turn of events, I tried shifting from one gear to another, backwards and forwards, but no maneuvering would set me free. I knew I had to get some help. The Hardin farm, the closest one in the area, was about a half mile away, and I had no choice but to get out of my warm car and trudge through the deep snow to the house.

Huddled down in my coat and shivering and numb with cold from the wind and blowing snow, I finally got to the big, two-story farm house and knocked on the front door. No answer. I knocked again and finally Mrs. Hardin opened the door and amazed at seeing me—like an apparition, out of the storm—gasped and with sincere concern in her voice exclaimed, "For Heaven's sake, Doctor, come in out of the cold." She took me by the arm and hurried me through the hallway and on into the warm, friendly kitchen. In less than a minute she handed me a cup of steaming hot coffee and added, "Drink that, it will warm you up." And then, without a second's hesitation, she turned and headed toward the back door and without looking back, she said, "I'll go call Lace. He's at the barn feeding the cattle."

I explained my predicament to Lace. Pondering just a few seconds he said, "Doc, drink your coffee and get warm. I'll go get the mules and get you pulled out of the hole in no time at all." Buttoning his coat and turning his coat collar up to turn the cold bitter wind, he headed back to the barn and in short order he came back with two big sorrel mules. Lace said, "Doc, climb up on old Barney and we'll ride down the road to your car." I rode Barney, Lace was on the other mule, Sam. Together we rode through my foot tracks in the snow the long, cold, windy half mile back to my car. We got off the mules and Lace hooked a chain to the double tree on the mule's harness, the other end to my car bumper and, sure enough, Sam and Barney, with my car motor's help and Lace's directions, pulled me out of that hole with little effort. Lace headed back to the barn with his mules and I followed him in the car. When we got to the house I offered to pay for the mule service but he wouldn't take a cent. Instead he said, "…come out to the barn, I want to show you my two stud colts." I could tell from his voice that they must be special.

I followed him down the path to the barn. Lace, proud as a peacock of his colts and his cheeks glowing red from the cold air, led me to a box stall that housed two big and fat, full grown three year old stallions. They were good looking horses but nervous and skittish. One had a white blaze down his face and as I moved closer to the stall for a better look, the horse reared and with his mouth open as to eat me up, lunged toward the front of the stall and struck at me with his front feet! Only the solid oak walls of the barn saved me. It was very obvious that these horses were just like wild animals, cautious, maybe even frightened by me as a stranger. They were on the defensive with every breath they took! Backing away from the front of the stall, I asked Lace where he bought them. Glowing even more with pride he almost shouted, "Bought 'em hell, Doc, I raised 'em both out of these two old mares we have here. I ain't done a thing with them since they was foaled—not even halter broke 'em."

Still trying to recover from the stallion's wrath, I asked, "How come you let them get so big? Man, they're full grown now and as nervous and mean as they are, they are going to be next to impossible to break at this age." I'm sure he knew everybody broke their colts while they were young, even halter breaking them before they were two weeks old.

Looking me straight in the eye, and with the frozen cloud of steam from his breath almost filling the cold barn, Lace Hardin said, "Doc Martin, they won't be no trouble to break—after you geld 'em, come this spring."

That remark hit me like a ton of rocks in a spring land slide and I knew that some way I would have to do it, "…come this spring." Again I thanked him for pulling me out of the snow and mud and went on to my pig call down the Bear Creek Road.

"Come next spring," as Mr. Hardin suggested, I did operate on those two horses but that is another story which I'll tell later.

I got to the circus in Dayton, early in the morning and after handshakes and a "Gee, Doc, how have you been?" I suggested we operate as soon as possible so we could have the rest of the day to visit. After a short discussion, we decided that the Animal Top would be a good operating room. J.Y. gathered his grooms to help us and we were ready to go to work.

Dr. Henderson, knowing I intended to do a standing castration procedure, wanted to know how we were going to confine this horse during the surgery. I told him I didn't think it would be a big problem since we had so much manpower available. He looked at me—almost as if to say, "I don't think you know how tough this stud horse is." We took the horse off the picket line, fastened a rope to his tail and put that rope up over the steel spike on one of the side poles of the tent. This would work like a pulley and we could lift the horse's rear feet off the ground when we operated. With just a little effort I injected a tranquilizer into his jugular vein. My plans were made and executed. In my mind I had achieved my goal—I was about to be a circus veterinarian! A few onlookers were gathering and for the moment I was the center of attraction. I was ready to do my surgery.

Now here I was the specialist—or at least proclaimed to be—and at this point, everything started to go wrong. First off, the stallion—teeth barred like a snapping dog—tried to chew up the twitch and the man that was holding it. The stud was fighting mad—striking at us with his hooves and slinging his head trying to get the twitch off his nose. In a last, desperate head-shaking lunge, he slammed one of the grooms in the head with the heavy wooden twitch handle, laying open a four inch long cut in his scalp. Momentarily we were defeated. We rested a minute, sent our injured assistant for first aid and then tried the horse again. There was one man on each side of the horse putting his full weight against the animal's shoulder and at the same time holding and twisting one of the horse's ears. Another man was busy shaking and twisting the nose twitch while two other helpers pulled the horse's back feet off the ground with the tail rope. We thought we finally had him subdued.

Now, by this time, I had a big audience and I could hear people talking about the guy with the knife. I heard one man mumble that I didn't look too smart. Another man said, "I hope that damned horse wins!" I am sure there were more caustic comments but I was too busy to hear them.

I made the initial incision and the next thing I knew, the horse lunged, his front feet slipped and he fell with a crash to the ground, in spite of all my help. He was kicking and squalling like a wild animal. In all of the excitement I shouted, "Let the bastard up," and my help did just that. More mumbles from the crowd. I ignored them all. Now here I am, star of my own act, almost defeated. I took a deep breath, wiped the sweat from my face and very professionally finished the surgery. Maybe I expected some applause but it didn't come. After a few moments my not-so-praising audience walked away, some still mumbling something about the man with the knife. The now ex-stud recovered with no problems, but was always a mean horse. Eventually the circus gave him to some rancher for a cow horse. Good riddance.

That evening, just before the night show, a cold front passed through Dayton and with it freezing rain and snow. The storm hit with all its fury and whipped the animal tent until it almost ripped at the seams. We contacted the building manager and asked if we could put the animals inside and he told us he didn't have the authority to let us do that. He realized our situation and told our show manager, Tuffy Genders, he would contact someone and get our move OK'd. The storm worsened and we blanketed every horse and elephant and turned on the space heaters the show carried for cold weather dates. We prayed that the blustery, bitter cold storm would stop.

The snow and ice started to build up on the canvas and Tuffy Genders told us to cut the canvas and let the ice on through—he also told us to move the animals inside the building and he would try to make it right with the building manager. The wind was blowing a gale by this time, and the ice and snow put a terrible strain on the tent and finally, as we moved the last of the animals out toward the shelter of the warm building, the heavy aluminum center poles started to buckle. Only radical cuts through the canvas top took the pressure off of the tent and we salvaged what we could.

It was a tremendous show of team work, with no regard for the discomforts that came with the nasty job. After it was all over, Mr. Henry Ringling North, circus vice president and brother to John, the Circus King himself, came to the building and thanked everyone for their efforts. He motioned to J.Y. and me to follow him and when we were around the corner and out of sight, he reached under his coat and pulled out a bottle of bourbon and said, "Boys, this drink is on me."

I called Mary Helen the next morning and told her I wouldn't be home until late that night, because the roads were still ice and snow-covered from the storm. I told her most of the story on the phone and said I would fill in the gaps later.

In later years Jomar Farm was graced with more Ringling horses when the Stephensons, the people with the riding act called The Saxtons, went to Europe with the Ringling Bros. and Barnum & Bailey circus for their tour on the continent. They brought three rosinback horses and a trick pony to our place to board while they were gone. These horses were eventually delivered back to the Stephensons by one of my farmer friends in his open stock truck. They arrived covered with snow but fat and slick. Stephensons were delighted and after touring these animals again, they were eventually retired to Jomar where two of the horses and the pony lived out their lives. They are buried on our farm.

One weekend Mary Helen and I went out of town to a veterinary meeting. It was late in the evening when we got home. As we drove along the long driveway to the house, in the fading evening light, Mary Helen saw a nice white horse in our pasture field. From what we could see, she looked like she might be at least part Arabian. We didn't have a white horse and had no idea where it came from. After we got in the house I called my clown friend CoCo, who was now married to an Ashland girl, and asked him if he knew anything about this pretty horse.

In his clipped English drawl he said, "Yes sir, Doctor, I know all about her." He proceeded to tell me why the horse was in our field and what a wonderful deal he thought it was for the Martins.

He told me that George Hanneford, of the famous Hanneford circus family, contacted him and wanted to know if, "Doc Martin will take my white mare?" He explained she was a finishing trick bareback horse but years working in the circus ring had taken their toll. She was lame and now was ready to be retired.

"Doc, I told George to just drop her off at your farm." Then CoCo added, "She is an awfully pretty horse and I knew it would be OK."

Mary Helen and I finally agreed that CoCo meant well, but also figured out that it was one more equine mouth to feed. But—I guess, as one of my friends has often said, "That goes with the territory!"

That was twenty years ago. I never heard word one from George Hanneford. We named the mare Scheherazade, to honor her obvious Arabian background. She spent her long lifetime here. She is buried along with the other circus horses at Jomar.

THE TEACHER

The day Mary Helen and I met Dr. Henderson and Martha made a significant change in our lives. First of all, we became friends, almost like family, and in the next two or three years, we visited them in Florida as well as many times on the circus. Secondly, J.Y. seemed to have faith in me and my aspirations to be an exotic animal doctor. He repeatedly told me that he would help me any way he could to achieve that goal. He also told me I should never hesitate to ask, if I ever needed his help. He added, "I am not too smart about some of these cases but together, we can figure them out." Quite a compliment from the authority! He told me that all I had to do was contact him and he would find a way to get to Kentucky!

After one of our visits on the show, and our repeated invitation to come to Kentucky for a visit, he told us that he had to go to the Mayo Clinic for a checkup. We suggested that he stop at our house on his way to the clinic and we could visit a few days.

Three weeks later I met the 8:35 passenger train at the Ashland depot, and J.Y. Henderson made the first of very many visits to our home. On the way home I had a call to make at Claude Groves'—my saw mill friend—to look at a mule that was lame. This wasn't the same mule I put to sleep a few years earlier so he could "tack a shoe on the son-of-a-bitch," but a new, nice, hard-working animal that Claude used to pull logs out of the woods. On the way from the train station to Claude's house, I told J.Y. about the mule that didn't want his feet touched and the tranquilizer. He laughed and commented that mules had a way of their own and he respected them for it.

We drove to Claude's and, sure enough, as he had promised, he was waiting for us—standing in the doorway of the barn, mule in one hand, a lantern for light in the other. J.Y. and I climbed the steep hill to Claude's little barn. Together we made the diagnosis—my mule owner friend had driven a nail too close to the tender part of the hoof and had "quicked" his mule. J.Y. and Claude hit it off from the very beginning, especially when Henderson said, "Claude, that big old number ten nail almost got to your mule's heart—you gotta do better than that," and then he added something like, "is this the same mule Dr. Martin gave the tranquilizers to that made him try to climb the electric pole?"

With a verbal explosion he replied, "Hell no—that bastard's long gone."

With no regard for his clean business suit, J.Y. picked up the mules foot and said, ". . . give me those nippers and I'll pull this shoe off." Claude didn't quite know what to think of this man, a perfect stranger—all dressed up like he was going to church—pulling a shoe off a mule's foot, after dark, up on a steep hillside! Still, he never hesitated and handed Doc the hoof-nippers.

He pulled the shoe and noted a little trickle of blood from one of the nail holes. Holding the foot close to the lantern so I could see, he pointed to the oozing blood and said, "There is the bad nail."

I finally took over and cleaned out and medicated the nail hole and gave the long-eared critter a tetanus shot. Henderson was elated. He said, "Jackson, that's the first honest work I have done for a long time." I had my doubts but already I could see he liked what I did as well as I liked his circus work. On the way home J.Y. commented that he knew now, after climbing that steep hill, why we hill folks have one leg shorter than the other—it sure helped when we were on the side of these mountains. It was an old joke but suited the occasion.

The next few days were great fun for us both. I tried to schedule my work to make it interesting for J.Y. but there was no need for that. Everything I did seemed to absolutely fascinate him. It amazed me that a man with a reputation of being the world's expert on circus animals, a job that was the envy of many veterinarians—especially me—revelled in some barnyard when I cleaned a cow, or gave a dog a shot in the clinic.

This was really the first chance Doc and I had to have uninterrupted conversations. While he was here, I told him that I was getting contacts from people with lions and tigers and bears and other dangerous, hard-to-handle animals. I asked him for his suggestions and he said, "You need a squeeze cage," and went on to explain how it worked. He volunteered some ideas that would help if I would ever decide to build one. That very same day, I made the decision to have a cage built.

I told J.Y. I had a friend who was a master mechanic for the Ashland Oil Company at their big refinery here in Ashland. I went on to tell him my friend, Clarence Hoenig, was the person who built the beautiful show buggy we used with Terri's pony. J.Y. suggested we call him and discuss the project.

The three of us had our meeting and finally settled on a design. J.Y. immediately acquired another new friend, and he and Clarence spent many enjoyable hours together over the next few years. Anyway, Clarence engineered the project, and had one of his ace welders build the cage. Before the project was finished, J.Y. added his contribution with four wheels and axles from a Ringling cage wagon. Later he commented that these parts had suddenly become surplus when we needed them for our project. Thank you, Ringling Bros. and Barnum & Bailey Circus!

Our visit was much too short, and Doctor Henderson left for Mayo's and then on back to the show. In most of our phone conversations, he always asked about Clarence and whether we had started any new projects.

Some months later, Bucky Steele, an acquaintance from the Ashland Oil Company's Christmas shows, called me and wanted me to work for him. For openers, he wanted the claws removed from a full-grown lioness. He explained that one foot had been injured and she couldn't retract her claws. They stuck out like razors and it made her very dangerous to work in the act. He asked me if I could do that.

He also said he had a full grown black bear he wanted castrated. He asked me if I could do that too. I told him I could and told him I would get back with him in a day or two and set the date. As soon as I got off the phone with Bucky Steele, I got on the phone and called J.Y. and said, "Come quick, I need help!"

Henderson made his arrangements and I called Bucky and made the appointment. When J.Y. got to Ashland, we went straight to the clinic and examined Clarence's handy work. The cage was a thing of beauty, strong and very workable. When Clarence made it, we designed it to fit exactly inside a large animal operating chute that was built in my clinic. We pulled this cage into the chute and fastened it securely to the steel posts with chains. That anchored it and it would never move. Henderson liked the idea.

We discussed the surgery and he assured me that I would have no trouble. Doc Henderson told me, "I'll keep a low profile. You can do the work!"

Bucky Steele's big tractor trailer rig was parked in my parking lot and all the neighbors watched as he unloaded a circus cage holding a snarling, restless, full grown, female lion. They were cautiously fascinated. I was apprehensive, but knowing J.Y. was there to back me up, I tried to act like I was in command and directed and helped Bucky move his heavy cage wagon into the operating room. We pushed his cage up to mine and transferred the lioness into the squeeze cage.

In those early days, before exotic animal medicine gained more finesse, we had no specific drugs designed basically for use in these animals. Most of the pioneer work had been done by Dr. Henderson, and that was strictly hit and miss, trial and error, until he found something that worked. The anesthetic was a big factor. It sounded like an easy procedure—just get a rope around the lion's leg, pull it through the bars of the cage and give her a shot of nembutal in the vein. Nothing to it! He added, "Sometimes they sleep a long time, but I just keep turning them over until they wake up." He paused just a moment and then added, "One tiger I did surgery on slept for four days!" I hoped we could avoid that experience.

The lion didn't cooperate until we pinned her down physically, with poles passed through the side of the operating cage over her back. We tried for nearly ten minutes to get a rope around her leg but she would bite at us, roar and rattle the cage and jerk her foot back. All this time J.Y.—and his cage-building buddy, Clarence Hoening—were standing in the adjoining kennel room watching me through the door. They both seemed to enjoy watching Bucky and me sweat. A thought suddenly came to me. Why not let this old girl bite something and distract her attention and then maybe I could get the rope on her leg. I suggested to J.Y.—I was determined that he was going to help—that he take one of the oak poles we were using and let her chew on that. He finally came from his place of safety and picked up the heavy oak pieces. He said, "I wondered when you were going to do that, it gets their attention—that's the best tranquilizer you have!" He stuck the pole through the side of the cage; Mrs. Lion grabbed it and started chewing it into splinters. It worked—for a moment her attention was diverted. I managed to get a rope around her front leg and forcefully pulled it through the bars. Then all of the snarling and roaring got louder, even with that heavy board in her mouth. I found the vein in her leg and injected her with the Nembutal. In a matter of just a minute or two she went to sleep. It had been a hard battle. The surgery was easy. I removed the claws from the front feet and bandaged both paws. History was made that day, because J.Y. and I had devised a plan to help control the bleeding, which could be a problem with an intractable animal. Instead of dissecting the claws away from the toes, we used a surgical braided wire saw that when pulled back and forth generated a lot of heat and cauterized as it cut. It was a very successful method and I used it for years, never having a bad bleeder.

The lion surgery was over. I was pretty damned proud of what I had done, in spite of the fact the world's greatest circus doctor and his buddy, Hoenig the mechanic, were safely out of range, watching through the door from another room!

The bear was another problem. I had declawed some house cats and had some idea of how that went and of what I was up against when it came to the big lion. At least, I was knowledgeable about the cat's anatomy. But—I had no idea at all about how to castrate a full grown, four hundred pound, fat, slick, bigger-than-life, black bear. J.Y. and I discussed this before Bucky ever got to the clinic. He said, "Jackson, its easy. Its the easiest operation you will ever do." He proceeded to tell me exactly what I was to do. I listened, but wasn't really sure he was serious.

"Now son," a new term he put on me, "The first thing is to be sure that Bucky has a muzzle on his bear. I assume he will because he is a reputable bear man. Then you have him bring the bear into the clinic operating room—the same room where we operated on the lioness—and have him lay the old bear down on the floor. Steele won't have any trouble doing that." I could believe him that far, but then he added, "After the bear is down on the floor you just slowly reach up between his legs and gently massage his scrotum!"

I was beginning to have my doubts and said, "J.Y., you aren't pulling my leg are you?"

"No sir, Jackson, you just do as I say and you'll be all right." I had to believe him because, after all, he was the master of his profession in the circus department. "Now after you have him on the ground and you start to gently massage him, that old bear will just spread his legs and most of them just make mumbling noises like 'umph, umph umph.'" Henderson smiled as he tried to imitate the pleasure rumblings of a bear! I was still apprehensive and finally he added, "Have your syringe and novocaine all ready and while you are massaging him, very slowly inject some novocaine into the skin and on up into the testicles." I couldn't help but believe him. After all, that's why he was here—to help me. But once more I said. "Then what in the hell do I do?"

"Just cut him like you would a young pig."

I couldn't back down now and I told Bucky to go get his bear. Up until this point, he had never been out of the big truck. As he turned to go to his truck, I added, in a nonchalant tone, "Bucky, don't forget to put a muzzle on him." In about three minutes, here came Bucky leading a huge bear that was walking on his hind feet. The bear was turning his head from side to side, obviously observing everything in the room. Every time he turned his head, he would sling foamy flecks of saliva in each direction. If bears could think, I knew he was wondering what was about to happen. This animal was at least seven feet tall and towered over Bucky's five foot, eleven inch stature, making him look small. My God, I had never seen a bear this big. And then, for some unknown reason, all I could think about was Kentucky's hero, Daniel Boone, when he carved on the big oak tree, "Today I killed a bar." In a wisp of a second, I wondered if his "bar" was as big as mine! Then as sudden as the thoughts of D. Boone came into my mind, they were gone and I realized that my moment of truth was there. I was committed. I followed J.Y.'s direction to the letter.

"Bucky, lay him down". He did and at the same time I watched J.Y. and Clarence move out of the way, to a safer place behind the big steel squeeze cage.

"Doc, this is a nice gentle bear and I have him under complete control so don't you have a worry about that." Bucky's words did ease a little of the apprehension, but I couldn't help but wonder just what that four hundred pound, seven foot tall bear would do when I stuck the needle into his scrotum.

I did just like my teacher told me—I reached up between the bear's legs, gently grasped his scrotum and massaged him. Believe it or not, that bear spread out his legs and went, "umph , umph, umph!" I was beginning to feel a little better but next came the needle. Just as J.Y. said, it was easy, and in a matter of minutes, I had that bear castrated, back on his feet, and headed back to the truck. This time he walked out on all fours. I think that by then the bear had it all figured out!

J.Y. was right, it was an easy operation, especially if you have the security of a steel cage between you and the patient.

Henderson was a good teacher. I was learning fast.

I can't let this go without adding something about J.Y.'s background and his family.

J.Y. Henderson was born and raised close to Kerrville, Texas, on a cow and goat ranch. He could ride a horse nearly before he could walk. Like me, he always wanted to be a veterinarian and, like me, he had a sincere love for a horse.

After graduation from Texas A & M College of Veterinary Medicine, he worked for a veterinarian in Shreveport, Louisiana, doing what I did my early days in a routine mixed practice. As a young student he frequently visited the King Ranch in south Texas and was befriended by Dr. J. K. Northway, veterinarian for that gigantic operation. In 1941 John Ringling North needed a veterinarian for his circus. At the suggestion of his friends the Klebergs, owners of the King Ranch, and Dr. Northway, North called J.Y. and offered him the position as Chief Veterinarian for the Ringling Bros and Barnum & Bailey Circus. This started his long and productive career. So—like me, the horse took him to the circus!

His first marriage produced two children—Donald and Leliah, both successes in their fields—Donald an architect, Leliah a career member of the United States military. Circus life did not fit this marriage and, in time, there was a divorce and Martha came into his life.

To understand some of the future, you must have some background. Martha Henderson, before marrying the doctor, was married to Karl Wallenda, patriarch of the famous Flying Wallenda high wire act. From this union a daughter, Jenny, was born. Like her mother, Jenny also performed on the high wire and was very active in the circus business. Jenny's first husband was Alberto Zoppe. He had an exceptional bareback horse riding act. From this marriage there were two children, a son, Albertino—or Tino—and a daughter, Delilah. This marriage eventually failed and Jenny married a performer in Karl's act by the name of Richard Faughnan. Faughnan was killed when the Flying Wallenda high wire act fell in Detroit in January,

1962. After a long mourning period, Jenny married Andy Anderson—also a wire walker who worked with Karl. To complete the genealogy, Jenny and Andy are the parents of Tammy, who has continued the circus tradition.

Most years, while J.Y. was on the road, Martha would stay in Sarasota until the show got to New York and the Madison Square Garden date. Then, she would get on the train and meet her husband and stay with him for the rest of the season.

In the spring of 1963, we suggested that Martha leave Florida early and come spend a few days with us. In April she arrived in Ashland carrying her suitcase in one hand and a bird cage with a little wild bird she had found in the other. Martha had a way with little wild things. That little vocal Finch in its cage graced our kitchen for several days. We had a wonderful visit and this trip was the true bonding point of our relationship.

Martha constantly talked about her grandchildren and what nice kids they were. She praised Tino and affectionately talked about younger Delilah. She expressed a sincere desire that neither of them follow the circus.

In June of the same year Tino and Delilah moved in with us. They stayed from the first of June until the end of August. Tino went to the clinic every day with me, and Delilah spent her entire waking hours trying to make Mary Helen happy. It seemed as though we had a new little girl and came to feel Delilah adopted my wife as a second mother. I recall one time when she wandered through our fields picking wild flowers, just for Mary Helen. She brought those few little scraggly flowers into the house and I helped her put them in some water so they would stay fresh. She was so proud of that. The children spent that summer with us and when they left to go back to their real home, parents and school, Tino was determined to become a veterinarian, "just like 'Vatti' J.Y. and Doc Martin." Delilah never told us what she wanted.

The kids were brought back to us the next year and we really looked forward to a summer with them again. One of my hobbies was the tight wire. I had a low practice wire and spent some time every day on the wire, perhaps dreaming that I could be a star performer! But alas, I could manage to stay on the wire, but I never became very adept at it.

Tino and Delilah watched me struggle and once bragged that they were Wallendas—they could walk the wire! It was comical to watch them as they tried to prove their Wallenda inheritance. Time after time, and no matter how hard they both worked at it, they just couldn't do it. At that stage in their life they were far from wire walkers!

Later—in August, Jenny and her husband Andy, who had a wire act, stopped in for a short visit between their bookings. They kidded the children and chided them that they would never be Wallendas if they didn't do better. They remarked, "Even Doc Martin is better on the wire than you are!"

The years went by, and the Zoppe children and Jenny and Andy and the Hendersons were often our house guests, or we were theirs in Florida. Tino grew into manhood, married and is the leader of his own high wire act. He is very successful, and long ago gave up aspirations of being a veterinarian. Little Delilah also is married and she and her husband, Terry Troffer, believe it or not, also have a high wire act and are continuing the Wallenda tradition.

Tino and Delilah both are "sky walkers." They thrill people with their solo wire walks high above the ground often over long distances, sometimes between high buildings or high over stadiums. When I watch them in the news reports or on video tapes they send us, I can't help but remember those pleasant days in our front yard, when they first climbed up on a wire that was only one foot off of the ground, determined to some day add to the Wallenda saga.

As these bonds increased and their family and ours almost became one, J.Y. told me that he would like to leave the nomad circus existence and settle down. I invited him to move to Kentucky and practice with me. We planned this at length but circumstances prevented it from ever happening—for better or worse, who knows?

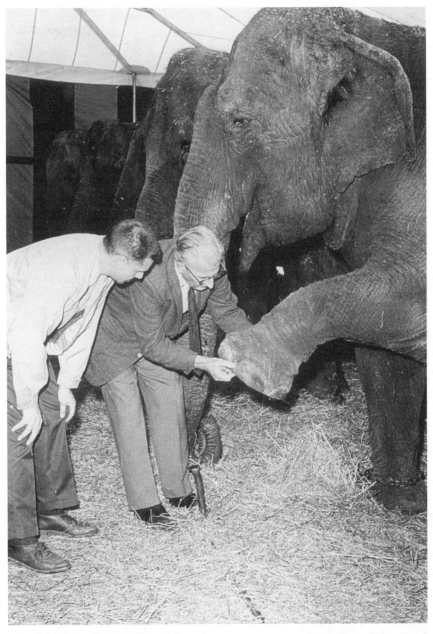

Dr. Martin and Dr. Henderson examine a Ringling Bros. and Barnum & Bailey Circus elephant with a foot problem caused by lack of moisture to maintain the animal's feet. The circus used this photo to show they carried two veterinarians with them that year.

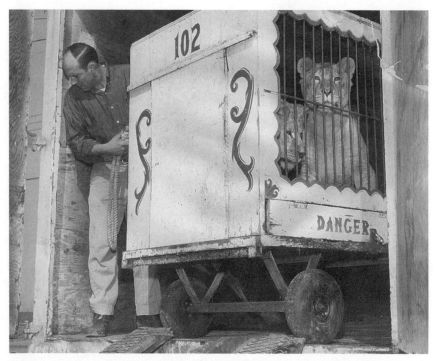

Bucky Steele unloading some lions for treatment at the clinic.

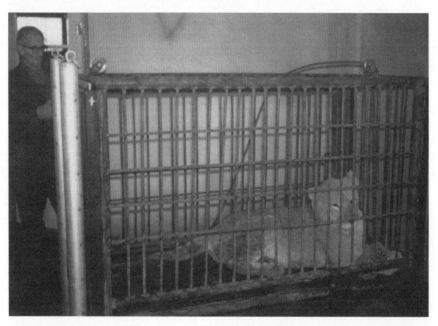

Steele's lioness in the special squeeze cage at the Martin clinic ready to be checked by Dr. Henderson for a deformed toe and nail before corrective surgery.

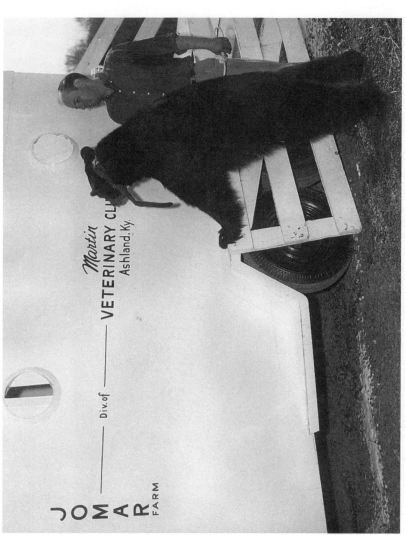

Bucky Steele and the bear that said "umph, umph, umph!" under the hand of Dr. Martin before special surgery.

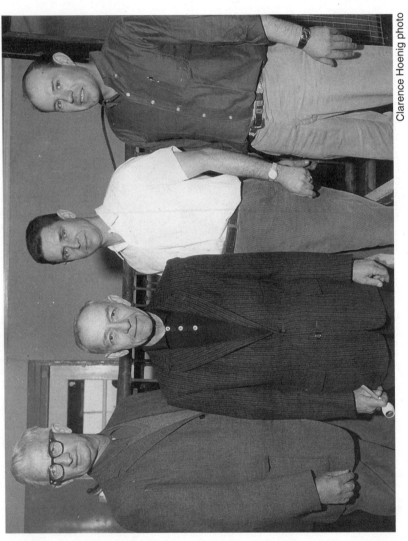

Dr. J.Y. Henderson, Clarence Hoenig, squeeze cage builder, Dr. John Martin, and Bucky Steele at the Martin clinic.

THE BIG ONE

Every person involved in our kind of show business knows what show you are talking about when you refer to The Big One. In 1880 the young Ringling brothers started a variety show. In the beginning they were their own actors and performers. In 1882 they took out their first road show under the title of The Ringling Brothers Classic and Comic Concert Company. The show underwent many changes over the years and eventually grew to a major American circus competing with the Barnum & Bailey Circus and the Sells Brothers Circus. In 1907 John Ringling bought the Barnum & Bailey show and title. The Ringling family also bought the Forepaugh-Sells Circus. In 1919 John Ringling combined these shows and the Ringling Bros. and Barnum & Bailey Circus was born. This was the big one! Over the years most performers aspire to be on this circus, as it is just what their logo says, "The Greatest Show On Earth."

My experiences with the Ringling Bros. and Barnum & Bailey Circus was an exciting time. I was never a full time employee of the circus but was paid when they asked me to do specific jobs. I visited and worked for J. Y. and the Ringling Circus for seven years—or at least that is how long I carried my circus ID Card. I operated out of my office in Kentucky but was on call to Dr. Henderson or the circus management at all times. I never knew when I would be called or what the call would bring—be assured though, each was exciting. I worked most of the cast coast dates including Baltimore, Washington, DC; Canton, Cleveland, Cincinnati and Toledo, Ohio; Indianapolis; Louisville, Frankfort and Lexington, Kentucky; Nashville, Raleigh, Winston Salem, New York City and all of the Florida dates and some more cities I can't remember.

During these years Dr. Henderson and I experienced a lot of things on the circus road that we considered routine and a normal way of doing business, but perhaps it wasn't very "normal."

October was a beautiful month in the Upper Peninsula of Michigan. The fall foliage was absolutely breathtaking, with brilliant colors. This was my vacation spot, and every year I spent most of this pretty month in the UP hunting grouse and fishing for salmon. I was completely divorced from veterinary medicine during these holidays. My hunting partner, also a Kentuckian, and I stayed at the same hunting lodge year after year and if anyone needed me, there was a phone at the lodge where I could be reached

Sure enough, one evening I got a call—clear up in the north woods—from the Ringling office to come to work in Chicago. I was to examine the animals, do what tests were necessary and prepare the health certificates so the show could move into Canada. Federal Health certificates had to be exact or they would not be honored. They were required not only for the Canadian visits, but for each state as well. This was my main job for the circus and I was frequently called to prepare these papers. The horses and ponies all had to have blood tests—so did the zebras, camels and llamas. Every animal: dogs, big cats and the elephants had to be listed on the health certificate by species. The horses were no problem, but just try to bleed a reluctant, mean, kicking, biting zebra, or a nasty spitting camel! I booked a flight and flew to the Windy City, did my work and in a few days was back following my bird dog and enjoying my vacation. This kind of work was routine, but all circus work wasn't so mundane.

One late summer afternoon I received a telephone call from the veterinarian at the Toledo, Ohio, zoo. This doctor told me that he had a small animal practice in Toledo, but also had a contract for veterinary services at the zoo. He informed me in very broken English that he was a graduate of a veterinary college in Europe. He was soliciting my help in diagnosing and treating some sick zebras. Then, as an afterthought, he said he had a health problem with a giraffe and wondered if I could help him with that matter too. I asked him where he had heard about me and he replied, "A drug salesman told me that you are the best hoof stock man in the business." My ego was inflated—I agreed to come to his zoo.

But I just happened to have an ace in the hole in this hand because the Ringling circus was scheduled to be in Toledo later in the month. I suggested we make our appointment while the show was there, and since he was entrusted to the animal care in this fine zoo, I would see to it that Dr. Henderson would come with me. I explained who J.Y. was and he would have the advantage of our combined services. Certainly a man of his importance deserved the very best. Now his ego was inflated!

On the appointed day J.Y. and I went to the zoo to see our man. This was a beautiful zoo, recently built and modern in every way. It had a fantastic marine exhibit and each display obviously had been well planned. If our veterinarian friend had anything to do with this, he certainly deserved a fine compliment! He gave us the grand tour and finally took us to see his zebra herd.

There must have been twenty or twenty-five animals in this group. They were in prime shape, fat, sleek and from outward appearances, seemed to be healthy. They were confined in a large area of perhaps five or six acres. A few trees offered some shade around the perimeter of the compound and, in the back of the lot, were some sheltering buildings out of sight of the viewing public.

The zoo veterinarian explained that everything was OK until the herd got excited and ran. Once they started running, several of them would stagger and fall to the ground. After explaining their symptoms the doctor told his helpers to make them run. They shouted and clapped their hands and one man pounded on an empty gasoline drum to make noise. The striped animals were startled and began to stampede around their large lot. We watched them run and, sure enough, about the time they had circled the compound once, several of them staggered and they started to fall down.

J.Y. and I looked at each other and right away we both agreed the zebras were suffering from strongiloidosis. A big word—yes, a rare disease—no. Our horse background solved the case. This condition is fairly common in horses. It is the result of an intestinal parasite whose larval forms migrate and adhere to the blood vessel walls in the rear legs. This reduces the size of the vessel and restricts the blood flow to a limb or body part. With strenuous exercise, the zebra's muscles soon ran out of oxygen caused by the inadequate blood supply and they ceased to function. Then the animal would fall down. In a very short amount of time, freshly oxygenated blood would find its way to the leg muscles and then the zebras would be OK. We questioned him about his horse experience and he told us that he had never treated horses and knew very little about them! Dr. Henderson and I never heard of a veterinarian who had not been trained in horse medicine! We suggested he worm the entire herd—we didn't tell him how to handle those biting, kicking, mean striped zebras—and gradually replace the affected animals with young, parasite-free specimens. We also suggested a continuous parasite control program. The last we heard was that after three years he had his problem solved.

After we solved his zebra problem, he took us to a large corral and showed us his giraffe. This graceful animal needed his feet trimmed. His hooves had grown long and curled up like sled runners. He was mean and dangerous and man shy when you got in the compound with him. It was impossible to confine him in a normal box stall. The zoo people built a squeeze cage that also was designed as his dining room, and because he was fed there every day, he soon walked into this trap with no hesitation. They intended to tranquilize the animal and then, with tree pruners, trim his hooves. It sounded like a good idea, but someone said they heard tranquilizers didn't work in a giraffe. He told his story to the drug salesman and the salesman told him to call me because I would know how to handle the giraffe. This is how I got this case. We examined the animal, agreed he needed a pedicure and we commented on what a fine squeeze stall they had made. Thinking about the zebra experience, we asked the doctor if he knew anything about these animals. He said no, but added he had thought about his plan and was sure it would work

We complimented him on his decision to wait and explained to him when you tranquilize a giraffe without giving him a muscle stimulant at the same time, he can't hold his head up and he is liable to lose control and break his neck. We suggested the drugs to use and the dosage and wished him good luck. He thanked us for coming; we shook hands and went back to the building and the show.

Some days later, one of my Ringling circus friends who was aware of my house call to the zoo, sent me a note. He told me a friend of his, a resident of Toledo, sent him a letter about a story he saw in the Toledo newspaper. My friend told me the story was about the local zoo veterinarian and his unlimited knowledge about exotic animals. A detailed description of the zebra case and the giraffe problem was explained and this doctor told how he intended to treat them and save the taxpayers a lot of money!

J.Y. and I got no credit at all—we didn't even get as much as a cup of coffee for our knowledge! Later on, when I mentioned this to another veterinarian friend of mine, when we were talking about the merits and pitfalls of charity work, my friend blandly made a statement I had heard before. "You know, Jack, sometimes that just goes with the territory!"

The circus was in Washington, DC, and just before the show date, J.Y. received an invitation for us to visit the National Zoo, a part of the Smithsonian Complex, and be the guests of the zoo director for a very special occasion—the arrival of the very first Komodo Dragon ever to be imported to this country. Dr. Clinton Gray, an acquaintance of J. Y.'s,. was the clinical veterinarian in the zoo and he told us to come to the back door of the reptile building. He said that the door man was expecting us. When we got there, our name was checked off of the dignitary list and we were directed to the second floor. The door man said, "When you get to the second floor, turn left and go to the end of the hall. You will see the other guests there." We did as he said and entered a large room that was filled with people. These were the most notable and respected zoo men in the United States and Canada! Henderson and I felt proud to be included in this gathering of dignitaries.

This room was perhaps sixty feet long. One complete wall was enclosed in glass, making a large compound. It was decorated inside to look like a jungle, complete with a stream of water coursing across the floor. Inside this enclosure was a large, wooden crate, perhaps twelve or fourteen feet long and thirty inches square. It was obvious that this crate housed the new giant lizard. The zoo's director, also a veterinarian, had flown in that very morning from Cambodia with his specimen. No one knew what to expect from the mysterious creature. Would he indeed be as ferocious as the natives said? Every precaution for the viewer's safety, as well as the dragon's, was taken.

The moment of truth finally arrived and one brave soul went into the glass display room and knocked the end out of the crate with a sledge hammer. As soon as it was opened, this man ran out to safety. We—the celebrity viewers—watched, not knowing if this critter would come out breathing fire or what! We did see, back in the long crate, some dark thing lying there nearly motionless. The absolute silence was finally broken when one man said he thought he saw the dragon's tongue flicker. J.Y. and I saw nothing. The animal never moved until the second day, and then it decided to slither very slowly out of its cage —a docile specimen. I guess if you are a zoo collector person, this is grand and glorious stuff, but to us it wasn't very exciting.

Dr. Gray did extend an invitation to us to tour the entire zoo facility as his guest. This is a state-of-the-art zoo. It proved to be very interesting to us when we saw the kitchens, the service areas and the veterinary facilities. These areas are not available to the general public, and for that matter, most visitors never give any thought to such places existing.

J.Y. and I were usually invited to visit the local zoos when the show visited a city. The zoo directors considered Dr. Henderson an expert and asked his opinions about treating animals. It was interesting to me that zoo work and our circus work represented two different kinds of exotic animal veterinary medicine. The zoos had no idea how to do the things that we sometimes did routinely, such as declaw a big cat, extract teeth from an ailing exotic animal or castrate some wild animal. Cosmetic surgery to repair fight wounds and cases of that nature rarely happened in a zoo, but our traveling animals were constantly exposed to hazards, if for no other reason than that they moved every day .

On the other hand, the zoo veterinarians generally were more scientific and their work was directed toward research and discovery. I like to think that this marriage of our work and theirs certainly helped advance exotic animal medicine toward the prestige it enjoys today.

Another year—1964—one of the King Ranch liberty horses broke a leg and had to be replaced in the act. J.Y. called and wanted Royal back on the show until he could break a replacement. Doc arrived at my house and, after a visit of a day or so, we loaded Royal in my horse trailer and headed for the nation's capitol. It was cold the week before Easter. We elected to go across northern West Virginia as that seemed to be the most direct route. Remember, this was before the interstate program was completed. When we got into the West Virginia mountains, we drove through areas of very heavy snow. Snow plows had cut huge passes through some drifts which were over thirty feet deep! After a long, hard trip we pulled into the backyard of the circus building —the Washington Armory —and unloaded the horse. He was tired and stiff from the long trailer ride. J.Y. and I were just plain tired from the strain of a five-hundred mile trip up and down steep mountain roads through the winter snows.

We left instructions for caring for Royal to "Repinsky Red," one of the horse grooms on the circus and a special friend of mine, and we went to the building. We had no sooner walked through the door, when a man came running up to me and in very broken English—he turned out to be German—asked me if I was the veterinarian. J.Y. chimed in real quick and said, "He sure is—just tell him what you want."

A big grin and then in despair he said his chimp had a toothache. J.Y. immediately spoke up and said, "Let's go, Jackson, that tooth can wait until tomorrow."

The man no doubt misunderstood J.Y. and he almost shouted, "OK, OK—I go get him."

I looked to J.Y. and he shrugged his shoulders and headed back to the office to report that we were in. As he turned he added, "Those guys will take advantage of you if you let 'em." He walked away disgusted, but stopped and returned when the chimp man came running back, leading a huge old chimpanzee, almost as big as I was. This man also had a pair of dental tooth extracting forceps which he waved at me and said something in German that I couldn't understand, obviously it meant, "Will you pull my chimp's tooth?"

"Jack, don't touch that big old chimp. He's big enough to really do you some harm. Let's see if we can get some help, if this guy insists we look at the animal tonight." About this time, two working men we knew came up and watched what was going on. One of them was a man whose only known name, to Doc and me, was "Pappy." Pappy had worked as a horse groom for J.Y. for several years and later, when I asked J.Y. about the man's last name, J.Y. told me he just never bothered to ask him what it was! The other fellow was just plain Roy. He also worked as a groom in the horse department and J.Y. didn't know his last name either! I was learning a lot about the circus.

The man with the chimp headed straight for a wooden chair that was in the hall where we were standing, and made the chimp sit in the chair and fold his arms. Directing his attention to Pappy and Roy, he told them he didn't need their help—but thanks. He spoke something in German—or maybe it was Chimpanzee talk, I didn't know—and proceeded to pull back the monkey's lip and show me a tooth that was barely hanging by a shred of tissue to the upper jaw bone. I reached for the forceps and before J.Y. could stop me, I grabbed the tooth and yanked it out. The chimp just sat there, arms still folded, and with a trickle of blood dripping from his mouth, looked like he appreciated what I had done. The chimp man was elated and thanked me profusely. I finally managed to understand that this animal belonged to Willie Kubler, who had just joined the show from Germany, and that

Mr. Kubler was in his trailer sleeping—he would personally thank me in the morning. What a way to do business!

When Henderson and I got to the building the next morning, Kubler was there waiting on us and did indeed thank me and offered to pay me for what I had done. I refused the pay but Kubler insisted then that he take my picture sitting in his big loafing cage surrounded by his chimps.

J.Y. just smiled and, looking me right in the eye, he said, "Jackson, you got yourself into this mess—now get yourself out."

Willie told me to follow him and, sure enough, he had one big trailer whose sides opened up making a very large air conditioned loafing cage for his chimps. He let them roam freely together and, contrary to what many chimp people thought, they never had any major fights. Kubler took me and we went in the trailer, where he sat me down on the floor. J.Y. was outside waiting for whatever was to come next and laughing hard all the time when he saw how disturbed I was. Kubler said something to one big animal he called Bimbo and Bimbo came over and sat down beside me! Willie took the picture and I got off the floor and with a sigh of absolute relief, joined my friend J.Y. Henderson in safe territory.

Now to those who know chimps, this would have been a risky operation, in the best of chimpanzee colonies, but Willie Kubler was a master trainer and had his animals under control every minute. Nevertheless, I was glad to get out of there, and never again did I volunteer help without giving it a lot of thought. J.Y. thought my apprehension was funny. I was thankful the episode turned out all right.

One last word about Kubler and Bimbo. In Sweden, Bimbo had starred in a movie and was quite popular. He was the center of attraction every place he was displayed and was almost a national hero. Kubler thought it would be the same way here in the States, but over here he was just another trained monkey. The act stayed one year on the show, as just another chimp act, and then went back to Europe— once again looking for stardom.

Elephants: No circus is complete without elephants. Generally the more bulls, the bigger the show and, if a show is to gain prestige, they get more elephants. Ringling carried eighteen or more every year. Some of them were "the good guys" and some were just everyday big cunning animals. I want to make a few simple remarks about them here. First of all, I am not afraid of the average elephant— just respect the hell out of them! Secondly, I don't dislike elephants, but I don't intentionally pet them or get too close to them, unless the trainer is there with me. I never forget that elephants are big, quick and sometimes dangerous. The nasty ones can hit you with their trunks and if you walk behind them, their tails are like baseball bats! I would never let my child feed one peanuts or candy. And finally, I have attended a great many of these bulls and have learned to really know some by their first names. Most are good and we are friends. A very few are bad and I avoid them if possible

Hugo Schmidt was, for a long time, the head elephant man on the Ringling Bros. and Barnum & Bailey Circus. He had come to the USA from Germany, first to the Mills Brothers Circus and then eventually to Ringling. He was one of the very best bull men in the world. When I first came on the show, Hugo asked me one day what I knew about elephants. I was very honest with him and told him that I liked them but the only things I really knew for certain was that they were very big, very strong and could be very mean. I told him that I would gladly be available, if he wanted to help me learn about them. For some reason, whether it was my frankness and admission I knew nothing about his charges, Hugo and I became very good friends and he went out of his way to help me. He gave me confidence and a lot of knowledge that very few veterinarians ever had.

Hugo had an elephant of his own on the show for which he received extra money. Her name was Targa—the same elephant which reached out for Mary Helen! She didn't have big soulful eyes or that little, elephant-like kindness look that some of them have. Instead, she was beady-eyed and when you approached her, she would stop whatever she was doing and look at you as if she had something on her mind.

On more than one occasion, J.Y. told me to be careful around her and not to get close enough that she could reach me with her trunk. He told me about the time he was walking through the building, carrying a ladder. He had to walk in front of the elephants that were chained facing a wall. For a reason unknown to J.Y., Targa lunged and tried to hit him with her trunk. Doc told me that by the grace of God he was just a foot farther from her than she could reach! He emphatically told me that he always kept an eye on her after that and even then, on two different occasions she tried to get to him! Hugo had no explanation for her behavior either. There just had to be something that Targa didn't like about Doc Henderson. J.Y. just made up his mind to stay out of her way and when he had to be close to her, he always had his eye on her. One of the first things I was taught in my indoctrination at Ringling was to avoid that elephant. I too gave her a wide berth until one day I was talking to someone just in the animal tent when suddenly someone yelled. "Doc—look out!" I jumped before I looked and as I looked back I saw Axel Gautier, Hugo's understudy, reprimanding Targa for trying to get at me! I had never as much as touched her or had anything to do with her, but yet she tried to get to me. Maybe I smelled like a veterinarian. I don't know, but I never, ever, got close enough to her for her to try to hurt me again— except one time I had been off the show for a while and was asked to come on at Charleston, West Virginia, for the Carolina stands, Raleigh and Winston Salem and then on to Baltimore. When we were in Charleston, the newspaper did a feature about me and wanted a picture with an elephant. Axel spoke up and told the newspaper man that he would get his animal for the photograph. We staged the picture. I was to pretend to give an injection into the elephant's shoulder. It wouldn't take long, the newspaperman promised; the photographer would click his picture and we would all get back to work. Here came Axel, laughing at me— you guessed it, with Targa in tow! I stood up just like I was supposed to, acted like I was giving an injection and when the camera man clicked his camera, I turned and walked away.

Axel laughed even harder and said, "Doc, I wouldn't let her hurt you."
As an afterthought: Hugo Schmidt died in the middle 70s. Targa was
passed on to Axel Gautier, Hugo's understudy. In late 1993 Axel was
killed by one of Ringling's elephants. As far as I know, Targa is still
on the show and I hope to Heaven she doesn't have some other veterinarian in her sights.

Invariably I am asked how I keep from getting hurt and what is
the meanest animal I deal with.

The lions, tigers, elephants and other exotics are confined and
cared for by trained handlers. Bears can be doubly dangerous if you
try to confine them. Chimpanzees are dangerous too. First of all, they
are just smart enough to think a little but not smart enough to remember to be nice when they should be. Confined or restrained, they
are savage —biting and grabbing with both hands and feet. I really
think I have more respect for the average chimp than I do for a lot of
the other animals. As a veterinarian I always respected the risks asso-
ciated with the performing animals while caring for them. This respect and of course, the expertise of the handler, kept me out of harm's
way.

Not every animal which has the potential to hurt you comes from
the wilds or far away, exotic places. The show was in Charleston, West
Virginia, and I was standing beside Frank Stephenson's Airstream
Trailer talking to him about one of his horses. It was hot and the two
of us moved closer to the trailer and some shade. I sure must have
violated some Holy ground, because just as I stepped into the cooling shade, one of Stephenson's wirehaired fox terriers Frank had tied
under the trailer, growled and snarled and lunged for my knee, sink-
ing every tooth he had clear to the bone! Convinced he had a good
bite, this little dog with my knee in his mouth shook me like I was a
rat! It hurt. Frank grabbed the dog and, of course, apologized but not
before he told me that this terrier was the meanest dog they had and
that was why he had been tied to the trailer just so he would be out of
harm's way!

We were playing Winston Salem and Charly Baumann, the

great German tiger trainer and star of the Ringling Bros. circus at that time, sent word for me to come to his railroad car and look at his little schnauzer dog. In his best English, interfused with a few German words, Charly told me the dog had an earache. That afternoon, between shows, I knocked on the door of the Baumann stateroom, was let in by his pretty wife and invited to sit and have a coffee. I accepted the coffee and then told Mrs. Baumann that I had some other work to do and I couldn't stay very long.

Charly called the dog and, as if he were directing a tiger to his pedestal, pointed to me. Expecting to examine the dog's ears, I had an otoscope in one hand and my coffee cup in the other when this little dog, at Charly's command made a big leap and bit me—hard— on the hand! I spilled the coffee, cussed the dog and tiger trainer Baumann all in one gasp! Charly grabbed the pooch, said some words to him in German and then turned to me and laughing out loud he said, "Doc, he even does that to me sometimes!" Baumann, the maestro of the steel arena and I, circus veterinarian, both put down by a ten-pound lap dog!

While I was with the Ringling circus I met and made friends with many fine animal people. I was interested in them, and when they realized I was sincere in my pursuit of quality veterinary care for their animals, they all helped me

Jack Joyce's circus career went back many years to other shows in early days. He was a great animal trainer: horses, camels and llamas were his specialty. He showed me many little things that helped me handle the animals and told me a lot of old-time remedies that I later used with success.

Colonel Trevor Bale was an animal trainer who came to the Ringling Bros. and Barnum & Bailey Circus in 1953 to perform the tiger act. He appeared on this circus on and off through 1964. Bale was a very versatile trainer and worked with more species of animals than any other trainer of his time, including elephants, giraffes, bears, llamas, horses, zebras, camels, gorillas, dogs and the big cats. In 1960, when the circus was in the turmoil of rebuilding after down-sizing from the canvas days, Col. Bale again had the lion and tiger act on the circus. He was most helpful and took great pains to tell me about the symptoms, ailments and remedies for diseases he had seen in animals all over the world. Even though his kind of medicine didn't conform with what I had been taught, I was grateful for this knowledge and, believe it or not, some of his little remedies worked very well.

Andrew Kirby came to this country from England as an assistant to Victor Julian, who had a very fancy dog act. Victor sponsored Andrew in a venture with chimpanzees, and from this came one of the very best chimpanzees acts ever to be presented. Andrew Kirby was a gentleman, a good trainer and a real showman. He had, among other things, absolute respect for the veterinarian even though he, like so many other animal men, had his own book of cures.

Andrew and his wife Marie became our very good friends and often stayed at Jomar with us when they were between dates. It was during this time I really got educated about the chimp, his loveable ways, his meanness, his cunning and his multiple personalities. Our daughter Terri worked with the Kirbys on several circus dates. I am indeed grateful for their friendship and this education. There were others on the Ringling circus who helped me when I was a "First of May,"—a term for a person who is a first-timer on a circus. Not all were animal people, but all were sincere and made my life in those days more than enjoyable and rewarding. I have utmost respect for Eldon Day, the money lender, time-keeper and husband of one of the finest ladies I ever knew—Peggy. They both took me in tow and made me feel as if I were part of the circus.

One final story, not about veterinary medicine, but about the Martin-Henderson friendship. The Thursday before Easter in 1967, I left the show in Baltimore and flew back to Kentucky. My trip had been rewarding, and on the day before I left, Martha Henderson, J.Y.'s wonderful wife and our good friend, and I went downtown to the big public market. She made a big issue of this market trip, and we spent hours while she picked out an Easter gift for Mary Helen. I packed the gift carefully in my luggage and carried it with me on the airplane.

On Good Friday morning—before I was scheduled to go to my clinic—I had gone to my barn and was riding a young horse that I was training. I no sooner got on the horse, when I heard Mary Helen frantically calling me—she sounded like something frightful had happened. I looked her way and just knew someone had died. In a loud voice, I shouted, "Who?"

"Oh, Jack, it's Martha—they just called from Washington and gave me the news. They want you back as soon as you can get there."

I handed the horse to my stable man and said to Mary Helen, "OK, let me go pack some clothes and call the airline for a ticket."

"I've already done that and your plane leaves in forty-five minutes." I went to the house, picked up my suitcase and Mary Helen drove me the ten miles to the airport and the beginning of a very sad trip.

Martha's untimely death demanded some detailed arrangements with an undertaker to ship her body back to Sarasota, as well as arrangements for J.Y. and me to get there. Martha was always afraid of flying and at J.Y.'s insistence, we shipped her body to Florida by train. We called the airlines and we were told there wasn't a seat available for us—the Easter rush had them booked to capacity. Cotton Fenner, one of the vice presidents of the circus, said he thought he could handle it and, sure enough, using his Ringling clout, got us first class seats on the first jet out of Washington on Saturday morning.

J.Y. was in shock, and since Mary Helen and I were as close to Martha as her own blood family, we too were, of course, very upset.

The next morning a driver took us to the airport and we were on our way. The train carrying Martha's body had departed the night before. Our seats on the airliner were the very first seats in the front of the first class section. We sat facing a wall, our feet propped up on foot rest cushions.

The airline people were alerted to our misfortune and the flight attendant made several trips, asking if we needed anything. Finally J.Y. said, "Jackson, let's have a Jack Daniels and water. I know its pretty early but maybe it will help calm me down."

The lady attendant brought us the drinks, and as we were discussing what was to come, one of us lit a cigarette and smoked it as we drank the morning toddy. It happened in an instant—flicking the ashes from the cigarette, a spark floated through the air and fell on the foot cushion in a space, not more than one inch long, that had not been completely closed by a zipper. Suddenly the airplane—at least our part of it, was full of smoke! The airplane cushion was on fire!

Very calmly, J.Y. looked over at me and said, "Jackson, which one of those glasses is water?"

I handed him the water, he unzipped the cushion cover and put out the fire. We never reported it to the airlines and often thought afterwards that we should have. It could maybe have saved a life, later on.

Three days later Martha Henderson was buried.

This story simply tells another of the things I remember about my times with J.Y. and his family. J.Y. retired from Ringling Brothers in the early 1980s. When he quit, I did too. I still worked for some of the other shows and private acts until I completely retired from veterinary medicine in 1986.

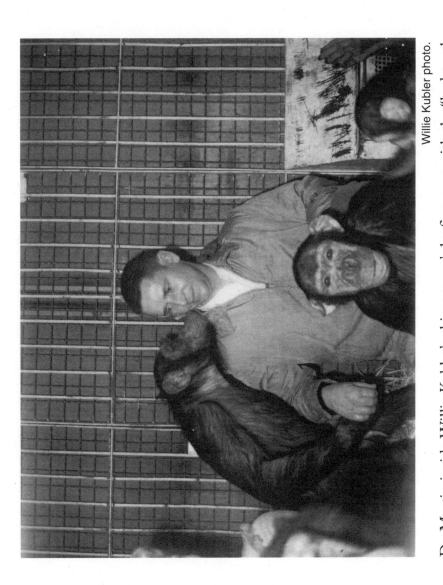

Dr. Martin inside Willie Kubler's chimpanzee's loafing cage with the "bad tooth chimp" (foreground) and Bimbo giving "the kiss" to an apprehensive Dr. Martin.

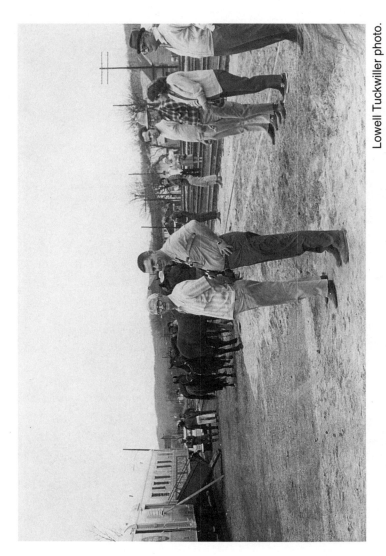

Lowell Tuckwiller photo.

Dr. J.Y. Henderson and Dr. John Martin watching as they unload the circus train.

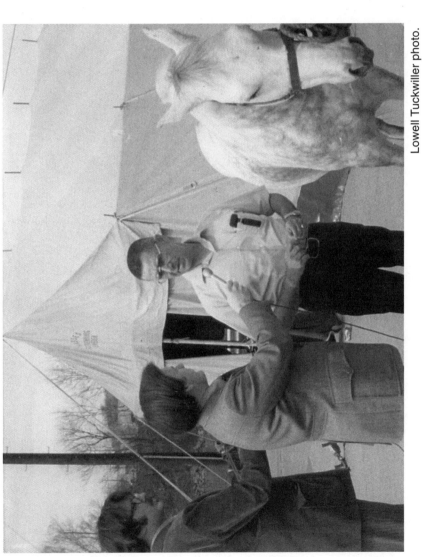

Lowell Tuckwiller photo.

Dr. Martin being interviewed by TV reporters while working on the Ringling Bros. and Barnum & Bailey Circus. The horse, belonging to the Stephenson Riding act, along with two others, was eventually retired to the Jomar Farm, a division of the Martin Veterinary Clinic.

ON THE ROAD

To the true circus fan, the real circus is in a tent. There is just something about seeing billowing Big Tops, canvas banner lines, flashy painted wagons and trucks that stirs your blood. After the Mills Brothers Circus took their Big Top down for the last time, some of the performers we knew drifted to other shows. One show was Sells and Gray, a title created for just this show. Our friends Paul and Chris Hudson were now on that show. Chris was a show girl and Paul joined on as boss canvas man and manager.

Early one pretty summer morning the phone rang. "Doc Martin, this is Paul Hudson, I need you," a long pause, "Anna May is sick—damned sick. Doc, she won't eat and that ain't like her." He coughed and then said, "When can you get here?" Anna May was a wonderful elephant on the Sells and Gray Circus. She was a hard working bull and a good performer. Best of all, she was gentle and easy to handle. Everybody on the show liked Anna May.

I asked Paul where they were and he laughed and told me someplace in Indiana! "Hudson, that's not good enough, where are you?"

He laughed again, "That was a joke, right now we are in Seymour headed south toward Madison. We play there in two days. But it ain't no joke, Doc—Anna May really needs you."

I told him the quickest I could get there was when they got into Madison, a pretty little town on the banks of the Ohio River. Just by chance, I had a classmate, Dr. John Lies, who lived in Madison. I promised I would call him and see if he could get over to Seymour. I also told Paul I would give Dr. Lies some suggestions since I doubted if he had ever treated an elephant. As soon as Hudson and I finished our conversation I called my veterinary friend and he jumped at a chance to do something besides treat hogs and cows! Mary Helen and I made plans and two days later—very early in the day—we were in Madison.

The lot was down on the river bank. There wasn't a cloud in a gorgeous blue sky. The grass where the white Big Top was set up had been freshly mowed and from a distance looked like a green carpet. The temperature was just right and a slight breeze was wisping just enough to make small ripples in the river and to cause the white canvas of the Big Top to float up and down as if it were alive. It was a perfect circus day.

I examined my elephant patient who now, after two days of Dr. Lies's treatment, seemed much better. I was satisfied and so was the show management. I thanked Lies for his help and left orders with Hudson regarding what I wanted done for further treatment.

There were two clowns on this show who were friends from our past and had been to our house several times for a visit. They were Bob-O and his wife, who clowned as Bobbino. Besides clowning on Sells and Gray, they drove the calliope truck and before the day's shows started, their job was to drive up and down the streets of each town— piping their music advertising the circus. Bobbino asked Mary Helen and me to ride along with them on their daily musical tour. We jumped at the chance and to the tune of historically familiar circus music, we wound our way up and down the streets of Madison. We were about done and had one more street to travel before we went back to the circus lot. We turned a corner and slowly started down a tree-lined street in this lovely old river town. Bob-O turned to Mary Helen and said, "Let's make this last street the best one of them all," and with that he fired up the calliope and blasted a noisy rendition of "The Gladiator's March." Even the limbs on the trees shook, it was so loud and blustery. Bob-O looked to me and laughed and added to his last comment, "That's enough to wake up the dead."

Suddenly there was absolute silence. Bobbino had stopped playing and was pointing a finger at a funeral parlor not more than fifty yards down the street. There were about thirty or forty people following the pall bearers as they carried a casket towards a waiting hearse! Quietly she said to her husband, "You and your damned big mouth!" Bob-O stopped the truck, backed it up and we drove down another street—very quietly back to the circus and my pachyderm patient, Anna May.

We followed Sells and Gray for three or four years and, thanks to Paul Hudson, I did all of the veterinary work for them, frequently traveling long distances to tend their animals. When the actual season was over, Paul worked as an advanced agent booking the show for the next year. Paul Hudson considered our house his home when he was in our part of the country. Later, after leaving Sells and Gray, he became the general manager for the Blue Unit of Ringling Bros. and Barnum & Bailey Circus.

In the middle of the summer of 1965, we were invited to Terre Haute, Indiana, to visit the Shrine Circus. The Clyde Brothers Circus, the show playing the date, was a large show with a lot of talented performers. This circus played mostly ball parks, fair grounds and buildings and toured most of the central United States during the year. Terre Haute was a very long day's drive from Ashland, Kentucky, but distance wasn't a problem when it came to a circus visit and we followed the arrows—a marking system used by the show's twenty-four hour man to direct the trucks to the show grounds—to the stadium where the show was setting up.

A lot of my circus clients were there, including Gee Gee Powell and her malamute and Eskimo husky dogs, Wally Naughton and his performing bears, Cemone the chimpanzee trainer, Karley Peterson, who was in charge of six baby elephants, and quite a few performers whom Mary Helen and I knew from other shows. Of course Terri was with us, and she found some friends from the Mills circus days, the Lacy Troupe.

The Lacy Troupe was a family act made up of father—Lotzy, mother—Lucy, two daughters—Suzan and Dena and a third young lady—Doris, whom the Lacy family had taken in. It was an outstanding act of precision balancing, where the five performers stood on large globes, perhaps three feet in diameter, and rolled them up and down ramps and through their routine with their feet. Terri spent her time with her old acquaintances and by the day's end came to me and asked if she could go with the circus. I told her to talk to her mother. She said, "Daddy, you talk to her for me."

The three of us had our discussion. Mary Helen said, "Absolutely not!" Her weak excuse was that Terri had no clothes with her. I argued we could send them. Then Mary Helen said that Terri would be an imposition to Mrs. Lacy. I contended she would not since "Lucy" Lacy wanted Terri too. Finally, Terri ended up staying in Terre Haute, off on an adventure of a lifetime. We drove home without her, wondering if we had done the proper thing.

The Clyde Brothers Circus played through Indiana, Illinois, Wisconsin, the Dakotas and early in August headed into Nebraska. Terri was watched after by the entire show and learned a lot about her friends and how they lived. Gee Gee Powell had the cotton candy concession, and it wasn't a week until Terri could spin that floss—show talk—like a veteran. She learned to handle the people and the money at the same time and really became an asset to the circus and especially to Gee Gee and her husband Billy.

One day Gee Gee had a sick dog. She had a dog act made up of arctic huskies and malamutes. When the act was announced, Gee Gee, dressed in a parka complete with fur hood, knee length fur boots and very short skirt, came charging down the hippodrome track, cracking her whip and shouting at her dog team as they pulled her sled into the center ring. It was a fantastic entry! She asked Terri what her daddy would do if he saw a dog sick like hers. Terri pondered a minute and said, "Daddy would probably check its blood for anemia. I think the dog's gums are too white. Then maybe he would give it a shot for hook worms." Then she said, "I think you had better take your dog to that veterinarian who is just across the street."

The dog was really in bad condition and was rapidly getting worse. Gee Gee took Terri's advice and went to the Terre Haute doctor. He diagnosed the case as severe anemia due to hookworm infestation! Terri moved up at least one notch in clout.

Wally Naughton had a wonderful group of bears that included a young polar bear. This little white bear was to be the star attraction of his bear act when it grew up and was fully trained. It got sick and right away he called Terri in and asked her what her daddy would do in a situation like that. Now Terri played this one smart. First of all, she had heard Dr. Henderson and me often discuss disease problems of the circus animals and she remembered him saying that bears were the wormiest animal he knew. My fine fifteen-year-old daughter said, "Mr. Naughton, your polar bear is full of big old long, white, stringy round worms." I don't know where she came up with this line of chatter but, I am sure, she managed it honestly!

Shortly after Terri had described the worms to Wally Naughton, there was a bear fight after dark and one of the older, full grown black bears managed to get to the polar bear and killed it. Before Wally knew it had happened, the black bear tore open the little polar bear and was eating on the body when Naughton found them. The grown bear had chewed out the little one's stomach and there, on the cage floor, were hundreds of long white worms just like Terri had described. She gained a lot more points on that diagnosis, which wasn't bad for a fifteen-year-old.

Mary Helen and I bought a camper and put it on our truck, and about a month before school was to start, we headed to Rapid City, South Dakota, to meet the show. We planned to make a tour of Wyoming and the neighboring area and then about ten days before Terri's school was to start, pick her up and bring her home.

When we pulled into the show grounds, Terri's reputation had blossomed. Everyone felt I had to really be smart for her to know so much about animals. She had earlier written us, "Daddy, when you and Mom come out here to get me, bring your medicine, there is a lot of work for you to do." These show people had a full itinerary for me. Only once in the three weeks did we get to take a few days off and see the sights. That turned out to be a busman's holiday as we ended up at the Colorado Springs Zoo!

My Clyde Brothers Circus practice started out by worming the entire adult elephant herd. This was easy. There were eight or ten bulls, so I had the bull man get two loaves of bread for each elephant. Elephants usually love bread. I started out with the first one and gave her a fourth of a loaf of the bread. She gulped it down. Then I gave her another fourth. She gulped it too. Two more fourths and she was reaching for more with her trunk. I really had her attention. When it was time for the last of the bread, I made an elephant sandwich with the big worming capsules wrapped up inside and offered it to my patient. She almost took my hand off grabbing it and gulped it right down. She was wormed! I repeated the same trick on every bull on the line and every animal got its medicine.

Karley Peterson was an animal trainer and a good one. On this show he was in charge of six baby elephants. It was his job to break them and get them ready for some kind of an act. His complaint was the babies had very sore skin. "Doc Martin, if I didn't know better I would say they were sunburned. I know they aren't though, because I keep oil rubbed into their skin."

Karley was trying to do his best with the oil but contrary to what he had heard, oil acts like a magnifier and indeed was making the sun's rays even worse. We got the oil cleaned off and put the punks in the shade and kept them cool with cold water packs. In a few short days they were much better.

Cemone wanted me to look at his chimps and thankfully they were OK. He had a baby orangutan named Oggie. This animal was the pet of everybody, and all you had to do to make a friend of Oggie was to give the little, long armed orangutan a milkshake! Then he was as content as a baby, puckering up his big lips and passing out kisses in payment for his treat!

After three weeks, our trip on this circus ended and we brought our daughter home in time for school. I often wonder what kind of tales she told her classmates about her "veterinary practice" on the circus.

While we were on the Clyde Brothers Circus two incidents took place that reflect a little of some of the things that can happen in this kind of show business.

The first of these happened in Terre Haute just two hours before we got there. Wally Naughton was going through a practice session with one of his young bears. He was trying to teach it to do the "iron jaw" trick like people do. In this trick the performer hangs on to a mouth piece and is lifted up in the air by the bear's teeth. Then Wally started the rope to swing in a circle and the bear hung on like a pendulum. Wally told me that it was not a hard trick for the bear to learn because he just held on out of sure self preservation.

While Naughton had this bear out of the bear truck, another of the larger bears managed to open the cage door and escape. The bear was free and as if he owned the town, took off running down the main street of Terre Haute! People scattered and the streets were deserted. Fear took over. One of the performers on the show was Cucciola. Cucciola was a midget clown who had come to our country billed as "The world's smallest bareback rider." John Ringling North brought him to this country in 1948 to star in his show. Since then he had worked on most of the shows and was well known in the business. He was a tough little guy and not afraid of the Devil himself! Without any fear for himself, Cucciola ran as fast as his little short legs would go down the street and grabbed the bear around its belly. He was hanging on like a leach to the big fat bear that was at least twice as big as he was! Wally Naughton running right behind him, caught the bear by his collar, snapped a chain to it and captured him! That evening when we got to the show grounds I asked Cucciola about the incident. He looked up at me and replied, "Hell, Doc, there wasn't nothing to it!"

The other incident happened when we were playing Scottsbluff, Nebraska. The show was set up on a race track at the local fair grounds at the edge of town. The night after the last performance, a group of the show people had a cookout, complete with big beef steaks and lots of ice cold beer. The party was a grand affair and went on far into the night, only ending when the keg of beer was gone.

Mary Helen and I said our goodnights and went back to our camper. It had been a long day and we were tired. The noise of the revelry carried on into the night and one by one the beer filled party-goers went to their trailers. We hadn't been sleeping very long when there was a loud knock on our door and an inebriated female voice bellowed out in the night, "Doc, come help us. We got Karley Peterson tied up to Gee Gee's dog sled and we want you to come castrate the son-of-a-bitch!" I was out of bed in a flash and out of the camper. Sure enough, two of the show girls—drunk on beer—had a half undressed Karley tied to the sled ready for me to do my surgery!

I woke up fast, thought about this bizarre situation a minute and made my decision. Then, in a very calm, quiet tone of voice I said, "Girls, I just can't do it tonight. Maybe we can do it some other time." I don't know why I said what I did in the tone of voice I did, but I sure said the right words at the right time.

Without another word, they untied my friend and disappeared into the night. I have seen Karley on several occasions since then and that subject never fails to bring on big laughs. After the laughs are over, Karley Peterson usually gets serious and thanks me for saving his manhood!

Both of these little stories reflect a lot about the circus and its people. They are devoted and fearless—like little Cucciola, when the chips are down. On the other side of the coin, they play hard and live hard but are really good at heart. Just who knows what would have happened that night in Scottsbluff if I had said, "OK girls, let's do it!"

Most circus veterinary medicine is a wait-and-hope-nothing-happens situation, but when something does happen it usually is an adventure. The following spring, Paul Hudson on Sells and Gray called and gave me his, "Come quick, Doc, I need you," story. This time it was Tommy the camel that was sick. Tommy was a show-owned camel. As camels go, he wasn't a bad guy. He would let you handle him and almost anyone could give him his commands as long as his routine wasn't upset. Tommy had a medical problem—he had a hernia on his side about the size of a grapefruit. It didn't bother him, but as a veterinarian I wondered just how long it would hold until he had a blowout which brought his insides outside. I had secret dreams of putting him on my operating table and doing a surgical repair. That never happened, but Tommy developed another medical problem that made him ill tempered and hard to handle. That is why Hudson called me.

My wife and I met the show at a little town in Ohio and the first thing I did was look up Dave Mulaney. He was Tommy's keeper. Dave was a friend of mine who had been with a circus for as long as he could remember. I first knew him on the Ringling show, then he came over on Sells and Gray, where we renewed our friendship. Dave worked ring stock, and lead stock, terms used to designate the performing large animals.

Walking across the lot to look at his camel, I filled him in on my tour with Clyde Bothers show and related some of the happenings including worming the elephant herd. Then I quizzed him about Tommy. Dave told me that his camel had another bump—this one was on the side of his jaw. "Come ovah and look at him, Doc," Dave drawled with his Massachusetts accent. "Something is hurting him—he don't eat too well and he's getting mean."

We walked over to the picket line and I examined Tommy and sure enough there was a large, hot and swollen, hard knot about the size of a football protruding from his right cheek. It was obviously an abscess, probably caused by a foreign body he had picked up in his hay. I ran my hands over this mass and Tommy's nice manners stopped right there. He swung his head toward me and spit. By absolute luck the short picket line rope kept him from getting his head around close enough for an accurate shot and he missed me. The abscess had to be opened but, the question was, how was I going to do it?

I toyed with the idea of just walking up and without touching or saying anything, jab my knife and jump out of the way. I knew this wouldn't work because, first of all, I might hit a nerve. Second of all, I probably couldn't get to the very bottom of the festering mass and, last of all, camels can kick and bite and spit at the same time. I wasn't ready for that. Recalling my story about worming the elephants on the Clyde Brothers Circus, Dave said, "Doc, maybe youah bread trick like you used on them bulls out in Nebraskar," his New England accent again evident, "would work here."

That idea sounded good to me. "OK, Dave, get us some loaves of bread and then let's back him into the horse trailer." Dave ran to the cook house tent and in a few minutes he came back with two loaves of bread. We backed Tommy into the trailer, pulled his head around to one side and fastened the halter rope to the side of the trailer. Dave gave Tommy a slice of bread, then another and then we had Tommy's attention! Every time Tommy made a move, Dave fed him another slice of bread. Then—I took my scalpel, located the bottom of the abscess and went to work. Puss and blood squirted out, the big mass deflated and Dave kept offering Tommy more bread. My patient never stopped eating. My surgery was a complete success. Mulaney and I congratulated ourselves on using ingenuity, which sometimes plays a big part in circus surgery.

Bobby Gibbs: A legend in the history of today's American circuses. Physically, he is not quite six feet tall, but as of late, is nearly six feet around the waist! A jovial person, with a well trimmed beard that is splashed with some white hair, he can be found scurrying around the circus lot, always busy, talking to a circus fan, or looking after his animals. Bobby is an announcer, a really great elephant man, a horse trainer, a camel man of good repute and a friend of about everybody in show business that I know. Bobby is married to a pretty Mexican lady named Rosa. She is as nice as they come and I am honored to be considered an acquaintance.

My telephone rang late one night and a big jovial voice said, "Hi Doc, this is Bobby Gibbs." He didn't have to tell me because I recognized that voice right away.

"Doc, I've got six little male llamas to cut, an old jackass—Rosa's favorite pet—and a full grown young camel to castrate. I'm up here at the fair grounds in Chillicothe, Ohio. I'll be here four days—can you come Saturday?" I assured him I could and told him to give my regards to Rosa. The town is in south central Ohio, about one hundred miles from where I live.

Just north of Chillicothe is a small farm community of Yellowbud. I have some very good friends, the Ebenhacks, who live there on a big farm. Martha is like our family, and her son Tom is almost like our own boy. Emmett, Martha's husband and Tom's daddy, died a young man. Tom grew up wanting to be a veterinarian like me. I vouched for Tom and morally supported him all the way through school and after graduation from Ohio State, he started a practice in Circleville, a town just north of Yellowbud. I called Tom and asked him if he would like to help me. He jumped at the chance and at the appointed time we went to the fair grounds and I introduced my young veterinary friend to Bobby and Rosa Gibbs.

We started with the llamas. They were small enough Bobby and his workers just held them, and I castrated the first one and showed Dr. Ebenhack how to do it. He did the other five.

The camel was tough. I put a rope around his neck, passed the rope along his spine and made two half hitches around the camel's body. I tied the camel's head to a tent stake and four of us pulled and tightened the rope around the animal's body so it put a lot of pressure on his sides hoping he would lie down. Now this trick works nearly every time on a cow, and I just had to gamble that it would on a camel. After a tussle and a few of my choice bad words, the rope trick worked. I made points with Bobby Gibbs, animal expert, first class. Bobby said he would never forget how I did that.

I scrubbed up the scrotal area, painted it liberally with an antiseptic and with a brand new knife tried to castrate that camel. I sawed and hacked, changed knife blades and cussed and finally managed to cut through the skin in two places and removed the testicles. I later commented to Dr. Henderson about this and he said. "Jackson, I forgot to tell you about how tough those old guys are!"

I saved the jackass until last, because he was the easiest of the operations. Dr. Tom, Bobby and I, and our help, took time out for a soft drink and after we had quenched our thirst, put the donkey up in a corner, rope in his tail and the twitch on his nose. I did my usual swift neat surgery and the next thing I knew, I had a handful of intestines! The inguinal ring was oversized and I realized the animal had a built-in hernia. Thank goodness Dr. Tom Ebenhack was there and, as I held the intestines up inside the animal's body, Tom gave him a quick anesthetic and the two of us, working together, replaced his guts and sutured him closed. I felt bad and so did Rosa and Bobby, but they realized that it was just a happening that no one could anticipate. The donkey eventually got well but they had to ship him back to their home in south Texas, since the strain of life on the circus route would be too trying.

One of the nicest shows, with the nicest people I have ever worked for, was the Royal Hanneford Circus. Tommy Hanneford called me to visit the show and examine little Ina, their very first elephant. Tommy and his wife Struppi pampered her like a family baby. Ina was subject to colds and sniffles, and Tommy wanted some veterinary advice. I went to the show, enjoyed the Hanneford hospitality, made my diagnosis and showed them how to give her injections. The last I heard was that Ina's cold was cured but she sloshed from the gallons of penicillin Struppi gave her baby. As far as I know she is still trouping on the Royal Hanneford Circus.

There were times that I didn't discriminate between man or beast if my knowledge of aches and pains was needed. I guess that I took some liberties and often dispensed my advice and some of my horse liniment and other potions to flying actors, tumblers and other acrobats for their aching muscles. Most were grateful and nearly every one of them was fast to say, "Doc Martin, we would rather have you doctor us than any human doctor we know!" Now I consider that a real compliment.

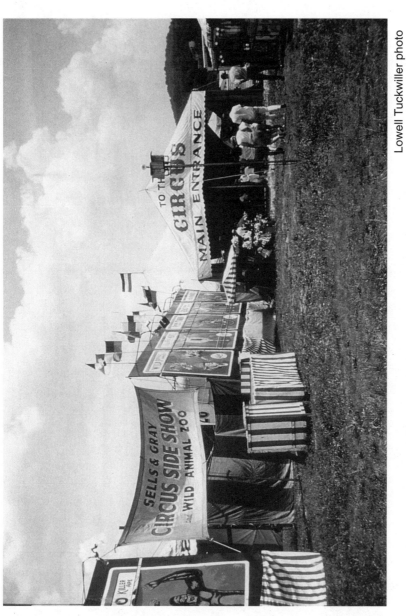

"To the true circus fan, the real circus is in a tent. There is just something about seeing billowing Big Tops, canvas banner lines, flashy painted wagons and trucks that stirs the blood." ca. 1963.

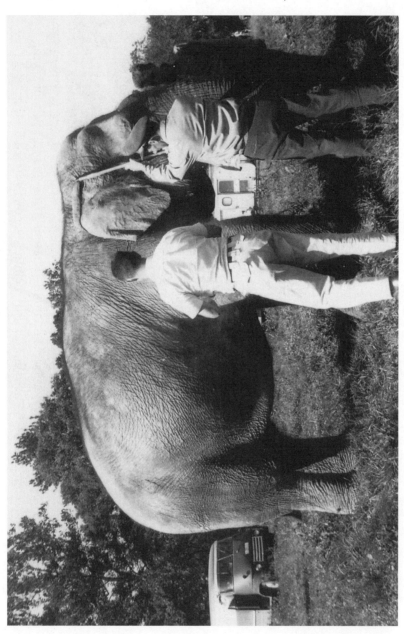

Dr. Martin making a house call to Anna May, a great performing "bull" on the Sells & Gray Circus. (ca. 1963)

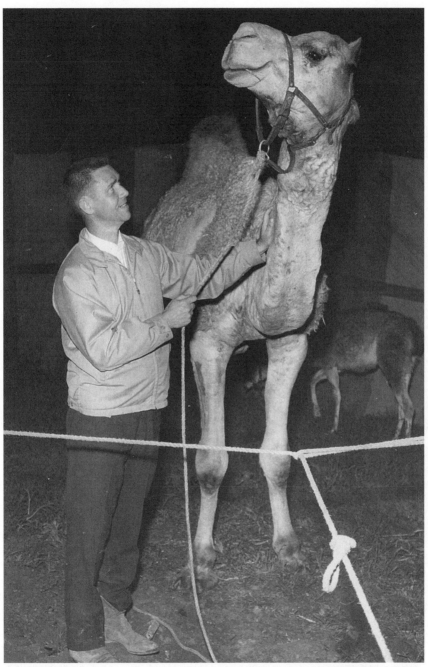

Lowell Tuckwiller photo.
Tommy is the camel which had the lateral wall abdominal hernia
and that big abscess on his jaw. Dave Mulaney and Dr. Martin
opened the sore in 1964 while Tommy had a "bread anesthetic."

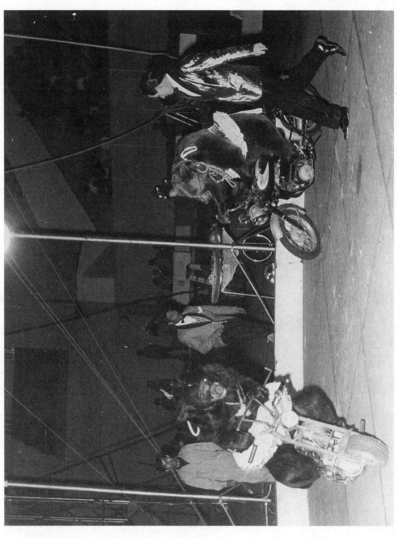

Wally Naughton's bears had a great act in the Clyde Brothers Circus about 1971 and were regular patients at Jomar and the Martin Clinic.

DOC, MY TIGER'S GOT AN ITCH

I like cats—plain colored cats, striped cats, spotted cats, big cats and little cats—all kinds of cats. I am absolutely fascinated with the large jungle cats we see in zoos and in the circus. These magnificent animals are the very essence of the circus and along with the elephant and the horse, constitute the vision of the circus in the average person's mind.

Wild carnivores are often misunderstood by the average person. Many people, including some circus fans, think these animals are tamed and are safe. This is far from the truth. John S. Clarke, an early 1900s English circus man and author, says it clearly in his book *Circus Parade*.

There are no safe tame lions, tigers, leopards or bears, and only a fool believes it. The big cats are fashioned for killing by stealth and with speed. Fangs, claws, muscles and sinews are to a cat what the cortex of the brain is to a thinker—something that goes on working in spite of temperament. A man who plays about with flesh-eating wild beasts is always in danger, however tame they appear to be, for the reflexes of an animal are quite beyond the control of an animals's brain.

In other words, they are not tame pussy cats!

Lions and tigers, and bears too, displayed inside the steel arena are often the highlight of the circus performance. These animals are presented by men, or women, who have the patience and the talent to work inside the big cage. Some cats respond and become good actors. Practice and repetition, patience and rewards—sometimes twice a day—make these creatures victims of conditioned reflexes. They simply go through the same routines day after day, being rewarded when they are right. Punishment is never used because that is the dark side in an animal's eye and fear brings on resentment and self-protection, which is what no trainer wants.

The exhibitor, or trainer as he is known, is often the show's star performer but is only part of the act. Behind the scenes are the grooms and animal caretakers including, on occasion, the veterinarian. My early experiences with these animals were learning experiences and thankfully, I had good teachers.

When Mr. North gave Mary Helen the American Quarter Horse, Royal, we went to the circus winter quarters in Venice, Florida, to pick him up. On the way to Florida we stopped in Centerhill, Florida, to visit Robert Baudy and his wife, Charlotte Walch. Baudy, a Frenchman and an accomplished artist, is quite a showman and dedicated to carnivore genetics and the raising and selling of exotic felines. For a period of time, he exhibited a caged act that was considered by many to be one of the best in the business. Charlotte Walch was also an experienced animal handler, especially expert with the large jungle cats. Baudy's cats had an eye infection and he wanted my opinion about them.

The Baudy compound is a work of art, designed to be a breeding compound and commercial center. It took much thought to design this establishment with its dens, shifting tunnels, sun decks and shaded cages. The tigers with the infected eyes were isolated from the other cats in large comfortable den cages placed in the soothing shade. I observed them carefully, and at Charlotte's suggestion for safety, I did not get too close to the cages. This is as far as the case went because there is no way, short of a general anesthetic, that you could examine, take samples to culture or treat these dangerous animals. Baudy, expert that he is, had no idea how to treat this infection. He commented to me that someday there would be a tranquilizer or anesthetic that could be used as a diagnostic tool in cases like this. I later learned, in due time, he was fortunate and they recovered without any treatment.

Other animal people realized the need for the same kind of drugs.

I would like to credit two people for their work in developing such drugs. The first is Dr. U. S. Seale, a Ph.D. at the Veterans Administration Hospital in Minneapolis. Dr. Seale was a scientist whose investigative work dealt in blood chemistries. He used animals for his research, and in turn his findings were converted to use in human medicine. Most of the animals he used in his program were Ringling Bros. and Barnum & Bailey Circus animals.

There was a tiger on the Ringling circus that was a "poor keeper." He just didn't do well, was sick at times and was hard to keep slick and fat and presentable to the audience. Dr. Henderson and I spent hours just observing this tiger and speculating on what could be wrong with him. Nothing seemed to help. The show was in Chicago and Dr. Seale, at Henderson's invitation, visited and decided to take the cat back to his facility and attempt a diagnosis through his studies. Transporting this animal was no problem. He injected an experimental drug into the tiger's hip, waited a few minutes for the cat to go to sleep and put him in the back seat of his car! He drove from Chicago to Minneapolis, put the tiger in a cage, gave him a shot to wake him up and then later did his work! Seale was a leader in developing drugs that allowed us to handle the big cats in a better way.

Dr. Lee Simmons, Director of the Henry Doorley Zoo in Omaha, Nebraska, is another person who was instrumental in developing suitable anesthetics. Dr. Simmons, a veterinarian, told me about the time he was moving the tigers from the New Orleans zoo to a new location. He anesthetized them and had all twelve sound asleep outside their cages, in the clean green grass, waiting to be loaded and transported to the new location!

With the advent of these new drugs and courses in exotic animal medicine in the universities, great strides have been made in my type of medicine. With the advance of technology, there are many capable veterinarians working in zoos all over the country. It is a far cry from the days Henderson and I practised our profession under the Big Top.

In spite of all of these refinements, I still resorted to what I called comparative medicine. I am sure this idea is not original with me but I think the term itself is. It goes like this. When I examine an exotic, I try to compare it to a domestic animal and wonder what I would do if it were a domestic animal. Most of the time it worked. Then, of course, the question was, "How do I give it a pill or injection without getting hurt?" I usually managed that too.

But in spite of all of this science and research, I stayed busy. The big cats would get sick and I would go look at them, practicing my own kind of circus medicine.

I was called to a Shrine Circus date to look at some tigers owned and exhibited by Pat Anthony. Anthony was well known and had a very good caged act. The history of these animals was they were itching and rubbing their hair off their bodies in big patches. Pat thought they might have mange. He came to me and said, "Doc, my tiger's got an itch!"

I examined the cats as best I could and would like to have had some skin scrapings to examine microscopically, just as we get on the house cats and dogs when we suspect mange. However, there is no way in the world, short of a general anesthetic, that you can do this to a tiger, leopard or lion. I wished then I had some of Dr. Seale's or Simmons' magic in my medical bag—but I didn't. I concluded since no new animals had been introduced into this group, environment probably was the guilty factor. I questioned Anthony at length, and the only conclusion I came to was the den cages he was using were not the cleanest in the world. I took my flashlight and carefully examined every inch of the cages. Outwardly they appeared clean enough but in the cracks and corners were layers of old dirt and hair. I took a chance and suggested to Pat that he buy some Sapona fly strips and fasten one on top of each cage. I told him to put them on top of the cage bars and wire them in place hoping these insecticides would kill the bugs and not hurt the tigers. I leveled with him and told him I thought he had some parasites that made their home in the corners and cracks of these old cages. I also suggested if he got someplace where he could really scrub the cages, it would be a big help. I wasn't really sure what was wrong with these cats but I knew some soap and water and a little parasite control had to help. I left orders for him to call me in three or four weeks and report. Three weeks later, to the day, Pat Anthony called me and reported I had solved the case and added I was the best damned doctor he knew. For once I was happy to be cussed.

Some of the cases that I saw in the cats were simple. Most were minor fight wounds that require little or no treatment. Once in a while a cat with a tail injury from another cat or a cage accident was treated. Parasite control was not hard because these animals were not exposed to any others and once they were parasite free, they stayed so.

The biggest part of exotic cat medicine is prevention. On the Ringling circus, and most of the other shows too, vaccination programs start in winter quarters and continue until a series of vaccines are given that cover all of the feline diseases.

Nutrition is probably the most important factor in maintaining the big cats. Only the best meat is ever fed to a lion or tiger. Bone is included and most animal men supplement the cat's diet with vitamins and minerals. Believe me, a circus animal gets the very best care in the world. The circus cats are content. They don't have to fight for survival or their food. They are basically parasite free and have expert medical care when they are sick. They live in a clean environment and seemingly enjoy their life style. They far outlive their wild jungle cousins.

Many of the sick circus animals were treated with homemade remedies by their handlers. Some called me and asked for advice over the telephone. Often they called me to come treat a sick individual or solve a group problem. However, the majority of sick felines were brought to my clinic, where I had the facilities to handle them. All of the surgery cases were brought to me except those minor problems that could be handled in the trainer's den wagons. The reputation of the Martin Veterinary Clinic and my services was growing.

CLEO THE LION

On a very cold, blustery February day, I got a call from Guy Gossing, the lion and tiger trainer with the Shrine Circus in Charleston, West Virginia. Mr. Gossing told me he needed my services, and wondered if I could drive up there and look at some sick lion cubs. It didn't take much persuasion to see a new show and get paid for it at the same time. My wife and I got to the building—this show played indoors only—about an hour before show time, and after inquiring from the back door man for Mr. Gossing, we found his big truck and trailer and knocked on the door. A loud shout inside said, "Come in."

Guy Gossing enjoyed a very good reputation as an animal trainer. He heard of me from some of his friends in the business. In the coziness of his warm trailer, we discussed his animals and his problem. He assured me that his cats got the best of care, food and housing. He told me that he had a new litter of cubs and two had already died. He was really concerned about the other two. I suggested we take a look at them and see what was going on. Leaving the comfort of the trailer, we climbed up into a big tractor trailer rig that housed the lions. It was dark, damp and cold in that big truck. A small light bulb swinging from an electric cord cast eerie shadows at the caged big cats who rumbled their uncertain welcome. In the very middle of the floor was an old metal gasoline barrel with a heat lamp bulb suspended over it and inside the barrel were two little tiny lion cubs, maybe five or six days old. They were thin and shivering, huddled together trying to keep warm. One of the cubs was nearly dead and the other one was breathing hard. It obviously had pneumonia. I reached down into the barrel and started to pick up one of the babies when the trailer exploded with a roar from the closest lioness—probably the cub's mother. I was startled. I broke out in a cold sweat! Composing myself, I examined both of the babies and suggested to Mr. Gossing that he take them to his trailer where it was warm and dry and we would start medicating them. My prognosis was not too good. I gave my instructions, left some medicine and he thanked me for coming. He also led us to the back door of the building and saw to it we had a free ticket to the circus. We enjoyed the show and visited for a while with some of the performers we knew and drove the eighty miles back to Kentucky. Considering this just one more case in my interesting career, I tucked it away in my memories and went on with my regular practice.

Spring finally made its appearance and one day Mary Helen was in Huntington, West Virginia, doing some shopping. In a men's shop, where she had gone to look for a shirt for me, a young man waited on her and after writing up her purchase, he looked at her name on the sales slip. He asked, "Are you Dr. Martin the vet's wife?" Surprised that she was recognized, she assured the clerk she was. He said that he and his friends were going to call Dr. Martin because they had a problem and needed his help.

This clerk was a college student at Marshall University and was a member of a fraternity whose symbol was a lion. The story rapidly unfolded and he told my wife that the boys in the fraternity had purchased a lion cub from a traveling circus. They had taken it home with intentions of raising it as the fraternity mascot. Well, the authorities at the university, along with the local Humane Society, soon found out about this and in no uncertain terms told the boys to get rid of their new pet. Someone suggested they call me. Mary Helen assured these young people that I would help them.

The very next morning waiting at my office as I drove in, were three young men guarding a big cardboard box that obviously contained something special. I got out of my car and introduced myself. Before I could say anything, one of them reached down into the box and came up with 10 pounds of scratching, clawing fury in the shape of a lion cub. One of the boys emphatically said, "Dr. Martin, here's our lion. Would you please take it?"

It didn't take long, after a question or two, to figure out that this was one of the cubs I had treated at the circus. As I ushered the boys and the baby lioness inside the office, I started questioning them about the baby. I soon found out that they had paid an exorbitant price of two hundred dollars for a cub that was near death and an animal that was surplus on the market. No wonder Mr. Gossing could afford to give us a free ticket to the show!

There didn't seem to be much of an alternative, so I suggested they leave the cub with me and we would work out some plan for the future. Three very relieved young college men waved as they left my parking lot. I knew I would never see them again!

Not being very creative, we soon named our new critter Cleo. She turned out to be quite an adventure in our lives, and this story would not be complete without her part in it.

First of all, Cleo had to be fed. I knew that this kind of an animal needed nutrition different from *felis domesticus*—the common house cat. I researched my books and put together a diet I thought would work. Part of this diet required bone and mineral not ordinarily found in commercial cat foods. Dan, my butcher, solved this problem every day with a supply of fresh chicken parts that included bony necks and backs. I mixed this with on-the-shelf kind of cat food, added some vitamins to the mixture and in a matter of a week or two, Cleo filled out, her hair slicked up and she weighed five pounds more than when the fraternity boys brought her in. Besides getting bigger and fatter, she was definitely developing a lion's personality.

It was obvious that she didn't like the kennel rooms and the dogs, so I started feeding her in my own private office. In a matter of a few days, I moved her there on a full time basis. To limit her access to the rest of the hospital, we put a fireplace screen across the door. The arrangement worked fine and soon most of the people in my town knew about the new addition. It did stimulate business and not one soul who used my services missed seeing Cleo, sometimes perched on my desk, when he or she came for a visit.

As the days went by, Cleo grew bigger and the screen across the door was made taller. By now we were cautioning people, especially children who came with their parents, not to pet the lion. We had a rule—look but don't touch. It worked pretty well. After office hours were over, and our day's work done, I let my not-so-little cub loose in the office and let her run and romp and play. We got to be good friends, and she trusted me and looked to me for protection when strange people with snarly animals were brought to my clinic. She also liked one of my helpers, I guess because he fed her. The other side of her personality made itself known when a second employee was around. She absolutely disliked this man and he was afraid of her. As long as they stayed away from each other the system worked. Bob, the one she did not trust, made it a point not to be around her. My wife and Cleo became inseparable, neither fearing the other and both having absolute affection for the other.

At times we took our little lioness home and she lived in the house with our black cat, Sambo. Sambo in reality oversaw our lives. He had been a barn kitten. One of the horses stepped on him and crushed his leg. It was beyond repair, so I amputated the leg. He was also a neutered Tom and was the first domestic cat I ever declawed. He was a loving cat and soon developed a better personality than most of the people we knew. Mary Helen and I wondered how we would handle the two cats together. We were pretty concerned that Cleo might try to hurt our three-legged friend. Our fears were soon re-moved, because when Cleo first came in the house, little old Sambo hissed and swatted at her and the lion ran as hard as she could down the stairs into the basement and hid! From that day on, Sambo ruled the roost and Cleo always watched the black cat with a wary eye.

I frequently took Cleo in the car with me and the two of us some-times stopped by butcher Dan's for our chicken backs and necks. By this time we needed several pounds a day. One morning, real early, I had Cleo at the supermarket on a leash. All the clerks knew about her and asked me to bring her so they could see her. The owner OK'd this and so there I was, talking to one of the girls while Cleo took time out to lay down and stretch in the warm sunshine that came through the glass window of the store. It was early. The store owner had just unlocked his doors when a car pulled up. The car door opened and a great big fat lady got out and waddled into the store. Taking a cart from the row, she made her way past me, Cleo and the clerk. As she walked by, I heard her say to herself, but out loud, "I think I see a lion!" Suddenly she realized what she had seen, came out of her daydream and yelled, "My God, it is a lion!" She turned and ran out the door as fast as she could, the manager on her heels, trying to calm her down. We both finally consoled her and after she was convinced it was safe she sheepishly came back in and I introduced her to my cat. That was the last trip Cleo made to the grocery store.

Cleo soon tipped the scales at twenty-five pounds and was truly a beautiful animal. She really wasn't much trouble but did chew on the furniture and, to this day, the scars are still there. As long as we didn't let everybody try to pet her, we just got along fine. One night, she hid behind the door and, in a lion's way, pounced on my leg and grabbed me with both front feet. Her big claws were just ready to tear into me if I struggled to get away. Instinctively, and not at all thinking, I kicked at her. With a loud squall and a hiss, she turned me loose and sulked to her corner in the office. Recomposed and ashamed at what I had done, I tried every way I could to make up with her. Nothing doing. Every time I made a move to pet her or go in her direction, she would snarl and back away. I could still bring her food and water pan to her but in no way were we friends. It concerned me that I had lost her confidence and her friendship. This standoff went on for about two weeks. I didn't try to make up to her anymore. The problem was resolved late one afternoon when I was through with clients and my help had gone home. I stayed and was doing some paper work. Cleo was sulking in her corner. I was at my desk. I heard her move and saw her stretch and yawn as she got up from her bed. The next thing I knew she jumped up on to my lap and was making noises like contented lion cubs do. Once again we were friends. From that day on, I was very careful not to push her too hard, knowing that her friendship was worth more than her wrath and distrust.

As time went by and Cleo grew bigger, I knew sooner or later, she would have to go to a home more suited for lions than my veterinary clinic. She created a lot of attention and actually brought in people who had never been to me, just to see the cub. One night, during office hours, a man brought in a sick dog. The man was obviously drunk and I was pretty well disgusted with him. I couldn't keep his attention and finally he got by me and stood looking in my office at the now forty-pound cat. Pinned to the door frame was a large sign which said, "This is a real lion. Don't touch or aggravate her. She will bite!" The man first looked at Cleo and then, with his whiskey slurred words, read the sign out loud. Turning to me, he made some remark about how he wasn't afraid of anything. Before I could say anything, or get him away from the screen barrier, he reached over the top and grabbed Cleo by the tail. All hell broke loose as the scared cat tried to protect herself. She made one pass at this man's arm and had it not been for a heavy coat he had on, Cleo would have torn his arm to shreds. I grabbed the man and pulled him out of the way while his friend, who was sober, helped me. The drunk was ashen white and scared to death. He held out his arm and said, "My God, look what that damned cat did." I reminded him that he had just read the sign on the door and he got just what he deserved. He was indignant. Stumbling toward his friend, he grabbed his dog and the two of them marched out to the waiting room and out the door. I felt sorry for my cat and I soon calmed her down. Several people waiting for my services saw the incident and asked me if I thought the man would cause trouble. One of the people in the waiting room was a lawyer and he assured me that I was OK, since the sign was there and the drunk had been forewarned. I never saw that man again but the incident made me realize that the time was getting close for my friend to find a new home.

The very next day I went to Huntington to see Harry Nudd, who owned and operated an amusement park. He also had a small zoo inside the park that displayed several animals including an elephant, some bears, monkeys, a kangaroo and two lions. I told Harry the entire story and pleaded for help. He said that he would take my charge, but to wait a day or two until he could make some housing arrangements for the cat. I delivered her there the very next day.

Harry Nudd was a very nice person, dedicated to a clean family entertainment park. His zoo was spotless and in a way unique. Inside the park was a fairly large swimming pool that had long since ceased to fill its original purpose. Harry took advantage of this and put his elephant in one corner of the empty pool and in the very middle built two big steel arenas. One was for his bears, the other housed his two lions. Quickly he had his workers construct a smaller steel area for Cleo. Here she could be next to those of her kind, but not be directly involved with the two grownup lions until all became friends.

Mary Helen, with tears filling her eyes, kissed her now big cat good-bye, and after thanking Harry went back to Ashland.

Cleo stayed at the zoo for over a year and, on occasion, Mary Helen and I would go visit her. I will never forget the first trip. It was Sunday, in the early part of summer, and the park was full of people. Crowded around the edge of the old swimming pool were hundreds of people, looking at the animals. The lions were roaring and the elephant trumpeted like a bugler blowing his horn. The bear cubs born in late winter were out with their parents and the entire display pleased the paying crowd. Mary Helen and I edged up to the fence and looked down at our now nearly full grown lioness. Mary Helen called her name. The cat stopped in her tracks when she heard my wife. Once again Mary Helen called out, "Cleo." Suddenly Cleo roared and jumped up against the steel bars and looked at the now fascinated audience. Mary Helen kept calling her and Cleo answered her every time! The people were amazed and watched as Harry, who had witnessed the entire proceeding, asked us if we would like to go down into the pool and talk to our cat. We sure did, and with Mary Helen crying and Cleo rubbing against the bars in absolute ecstasy, we enjoyed a tearful but perfect day. We went back many times, and as time went on Cleo still recognized Mary Helen and it was always fun to get reacquainted.

One day she got sick and Harry called me, wondering if it would be OK if they brought her to the clinic for me to look after. I told them to bring her on down. The handlers at the zoo had become friends of hers and they brought her in the back of a panel truck, secured only with a rope and a collar. This was enough, and they brought her inside where I examined her and started treatment. We elected to keep her a few days until she was well. Matter of fact, Harry expected this and had sent some lion food with her from his zoo. Now it was interesting to see what would happen. It didn't take long for us to find out. Immediately she fell back into her old habits. One look at my helper Bob and she became a mass of feline fury, teeth and claws. It was really frightening. Bob never went close to her again, not even to look through the door! Stormy, my manager, had no trouble at all with her and Mary Helen and I petted her just like we did when she was a little kitten. She soon recovered and went back to Harry's, only to be traded in the course of the zoo business, for two large baboons. That was the last exotic animal we ever owned. Certainly they are not for everybody.

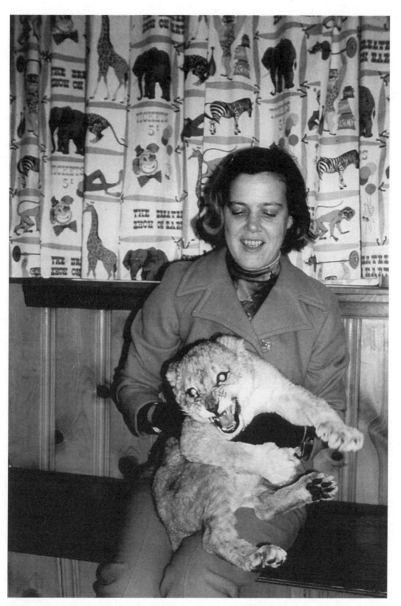

Mary Helen and Cleo, who is angry because Mary H. is unknowingly sitting on her tail!

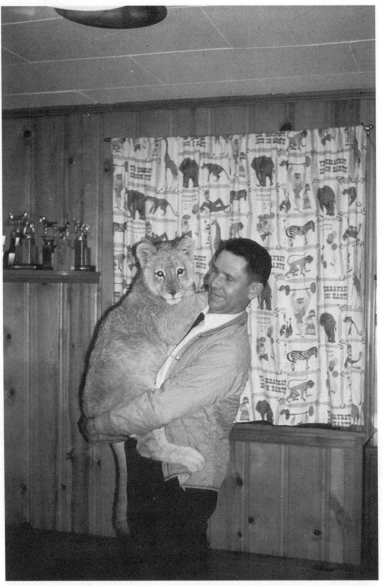

Cleo gives Dr. Martin an affectionate "kiss." Twenty-five pounds later, Cleo realized she was a real African lioness and was sent to a small zoo in West Virginia.

THE CIRCUS COMES TO THE CLINIC

Back home in Ashland, Mary Helen and I lived anything but a normal quiet life. We constantly had someone from some circus staying on our property. Charlie and Beverly Allen from California came one day with some bears and a trained zebra. The two grown bears were absolutely the nicest specimens I ever saw. They were well mannered—for bears—fat and slick, beautiful hair coats. Charlie also had a young male bear he was just breaking. The zebra was a football kicking animal and was, like most zebras, mean, mean, mean and meaner—that is when he had his bridle off! With it on, he was as docile as a zebra can get!

Charlie kept him in one of the stalls in my clinic barn and early one morning their hired man came running up to the office to tell me the zebra pulled his bridle off and was trying to kick the barn down. He pleaded with me. "For God's sake come help me. Charlie and Mrs. Allen have gone to the grocery store and they'll kill me when they get back if we don't calm that striped jackass down!"

I told him to calm down himself and asked Stormy, my office man, to come and help us. Sure enough the bridle was off and on the floor. The zebra had stomped it until it was nearly torn to pieces. The question was, how were we going to retrieve what was left of the bridle and then how were we going to get it on the animal when we did? I remembered Lace Hardin's wild stallions and got my lariat. Carefully, and after about five or six attempts, I lassoed Mr. Stripes and the three of us pulled his head right up to the door frame as hard as we could. His eyes bulged out, his tongue lolled to the side and he gasped as he struggled and passed out from lack of air. The very instant he went down, Stormy was in that stall in a flash and retrieved the bridle while the hired man grabbed the zebra's ear and held him down. I tied the rope fast to the post and, while he was still passed out, managed to get the damaged bridle back on him. And then I prayed, "Lord, don't let this animal die." We loosened the rope and in about two or three seconds my zebra took a deep breath, rolled his eyes and got on his feet. He was back to normal, politely chewing away at the bit in his mouth.

Charlie and Beverly came back a short while later and as they parked the car Charlie said, "Good morning, Doc, every thing OK here?"

The hired man looked at me and then at Stormy and before either one of them could say a word, I replied, "Couldn't be a better day."

They parked their trailer down on the lower level of the clinic and on pretty days chained the two big bears together by their collars with a very short piece of chain and then turned them loose in my paddocks to graze. They would eat grass like old cows and appeared to be just as content. I remember one incident that was really funny. My clinic was built on corner property and the bears were around the corner behind the main clinic building. It was not unusual to see cars drive by the paddocks and slow down to watch these bears eat their grass. One day I was outside talking to a client and I saw a car come speeding down the road. The driver must have seen the bears loose in the paddock, slammed on the brakes and brought the car to a skidding halt. He jumped out of his car, gawked at the bears and yelled for the entire neighborhood and me to hear, "Well I'll be damned!"

Charlie Allen's third bear was a little guy, weighing maybe seventy-five pounds. He was hardly chain broke and only Charlie could do much with him. One day he stopped me as I was coming to work and asked me if I would castrate the small bear before he got any bigger or mean. Of course I consented and in due time did the surgery. Charlie Allen had trained a lot of animals for the movies including the rhinoceros used in the *Dr. Doolittle* movie. After the Allens left us, Beverly continued to write to Mary Helen updating us on their life and inquiring about ours. In one of the letters she told us Charlie had signed a contract to work some animals for a new television show called "Gentle Ben." I like to tell people that the reason old Ben was so gentle was because he felt the wrath of my surgical scalpel when I changed him from a "him" to an "it," but in reality, there were several bears used in that series.

Many of the circus animals came to me at my clinic or my home. Our friends from the Ringling show, Andrew and Marie Kirby, had an outstanding chimpanzee act. They stopped at our house as they crossed the country from date to date. Andrew was a very knowledge-able person about most things and was, for a layman, pretty well versed in veterinary medicine. Nevertheless, he never did anything to any of his animals without consulting me first. I appreciated that.

The Kirbys had six chimps. A young male, Henry, was the star of the show, and of course Andrew's pride and joy. Henry was just like the other chimpanzees, just smart enough to learn and not smart enough to remember—and that made him mischievous and even dangerous at times. Another Kirby chimp was Suzy. She was the matriarch of the troupe and was full grown. Her attention to herself was amazing. Every night she would take apart the newspapers that lined her cage and fold them neatly on a little pile. Then as she laid down, before going to sleep, she very carefully unfolded them and put them over her for bed covers! Vocally she ruled the roost when one of the younger animals got out of line. The other four all had personali-ties of their own and made an interesting study.

Chimps lose their attention span when you are working on them. Marie and Andrew had a set routine every morning when they fed their animals and cleaned the cages. All of the animals were taken out of the cage and made to sit on the edge of a couch with their arms folded to keep their busy little hands out of trouble. Andrew would clean cages and Marie would watch her charges. It didn't take long before one of the monkeys—in this situation, a benevolent term— forgot to fold his arms and reached for Marie or the curtains or anything his mind wandered to. Marie always carried a stout stick during this ritual and when one got out of line she threatened to hit the chimp. There was hardly ever a blow struck but in a flash the animal was back on the couch, arms folded, again a perfect gentleman. By the time Andrew would finish his cleaning, Marie would go through this routine maybe five or six times.

Kirby's home was a custom-built bus, with the chimp room in the back and Kirby's own living quarters in the front. When they came to Ashland, they parked the bus in our driveway, plugged into our electricity and hooked their hoses up to our water and made themselves at home. Most mornings Marie would invite us to their bus for breakfast, which was a break for Mary Helen.

I was always fascinated by these animals and one morning Andrew brought Henry to the breakfast table to eat with us! Henry had on his shoes and some trousers and a shirt. He sat at the breakfast table with his hands folded while Marie fixed his bowl of cereal. Then, like a human, he picked up his spoon and waited for her to pour milk on the cereal before he started to eat it. Andrew gave him a cup of coffee and Henry took his spoon and got sugar out of the bowl, put it in his coffee and stirred! He was amazing. But Henry had some habits that weren't the greatest too. Like most of these animals he could get very mean and when he threw these temper tantrums the only thing that would get his attention was the sound of a gun going off. Andrew carried a pistol concealed under his coat when he worked the chimp act and on more than one occasion was forced to fire the blanks during a performance.

On a very nice morning Andrew went with me to the clinic while Marie and Mary Helen were baby-sitting with the animals. The girls were sitting on our front porch enjoying the warm sun when all of a sudden Marie shouted, "My God, Mary Helen, Henry is loose!" She was quick to add, "Call Doc's office and get Andrew back out here as quick as you can." Mary Helen ran in the house and made the call to my clinic, which was eight miles away.

Now, our home is situated on about two acres of our farm land.

We have many huge oak, hickory and walnut trees in the yard. In a flash Henry was in chimp heaven, swinging as only a chimpanzee can from branch to branch and screaming his delight. Marie was frantic; Mary Helen was frightened and ran into the house. Marie said, "Let's don't panic—let him play and when Andrew gets here he can get him—let's just hope he doesn't run away!"

Henry, perhaps tired of swinging in the trees, dropped down from his tree limb and ran around the end of the house and for some reason climbed up on a balcony porch that overlooks our backyard. There is a wrought iron railing around the porch, and Henry climbed up and walked along the top of the railing like a tight rope walker, balancing himself with his extended arms! Marie saw her chance and told Mary Helen that she was going to open the door that led from the porch into the house and maybe Henry would decide to come in. It worked—now the chimp was at least confined inside of the house and the danger of complete escape was over. Next trick was to catch him.

The scenario: Mary Helen disappears, Marie goes out the front door toward the bus for her stout stick and her gun and Henry strolls in the back door and makes himself at home. Marie told Mary Helen if Henry made it to our bedroom, she had him under control because he would jump up on the bed and fold his arms at her command. No one knows what Henry was doing while Marie was getting her war weapons but when she came back, Henry was sitting on our bed just as if he lived there! Andrew and I got home about this time, and Henry was put back in his cage. The crisis was over.

Then it dawned on Marie that Mary Helen was completely absent during the entire episode and asked her, "Hey, Mary, where were you when all of this was happening?"

A shaky voice replied, "I was hiding in the hall closet."

There were other chimpanzee stories too. Several trainers brought their animals to have their teeth pulled. A chimp will grow several sets of teeth in a lifetime and for safety's sake, all of the incisors are extracted, leaving only the molars so the chimp can eat. When these cases came in, I called my dentist friend Dr. Paul Savage and he came and did the honors. Paul was a great dentist, a little of an egotist like the rest of us, and delighted in doing something a little different. I would give the general anesthetic, Paul was the surgeon and the client was more than satisfied to have such a professional team.

There are heartbreaks in circus animal medicine too. Jerry Lipko, a good chimpanzee trainer and showman, came to my office one day with a very sick baby chimp. One look at the dehydrated, thin, obviously critically ill baby animal made me shudder at my prognosis. Jerry left the baby in my care and I worked up the case including laboratory aids and even a consultation with the local pediatrician. The final diagnosis was a probable inherited liver disorder that in no way reflected Lipko's care. My hospital staff and I did what we could for the sick little guy including twenty-four hour round-the-clock care, IV fluids, antibiotics and other supportive treatment. My patient died. In spite of the fact my staff was somewhat calloused at seeing animals die, it was several days before we could forget that poor little animal and how it suffered. One day several months after the chimpanzee died, I came to the clinic one morning and found one of the girls that worked for me crying her heart out. I thought she lost her lover or someone in the family had passed away. I asked her what was wrong and she looked up at me with her tear-filled eyes and said, "Doc, I was just thinking about that poor baby chimp of Mr. Lipko's." Now I call that compassion!

Most of the exotics we treated got well and went their way. Some were tough to handle but sometimes their very nature helped us and our work. I have in mind a rhesus monkey who came to me from a carnival man. The monkey had ringworm sores all over his body. He scratched and rubbed until he was bleeding from most of the sores. I tranquilized him, gave him some antibiotics and started rubbing an antifungal creme into the sore spots. Every time I touched this guy he would try to bite, scream and raise all kinds of trouble as most monkeys do. After three or four days of this fighting I finally gave up in disgust and set the jar of ointment inside the cage door while I went to answer the telephone. I finished my conversation, and when I went back to my long tailed friend, there he sat, salving his own wounds with the ringworm medicine in the jar! We kept this animal for a week and once a day put a jar of antifungal creme in his cage. Sure enough he repeated the act, rubbed the medicine into the sores and eventually recovered!

Not every pleasant happening in our lives was a medical case, but most were somehow related to our unique life-style. Our home life was often a circus itself with people coming and going. There were no typical calm, quiet days like most people enjoy. All we often needed was to have someone like Merle Evans and his circus band on the farm and we would have been in business. I well remember August of 1963.

Tino and Delilah Zoppe were spending their first summer with us. Dr. Henderson and his wife Martha came at the same time for a short visit while the Ringling circus was playing close by in West Virginia. That was fine but at the same time, Gee Gee and Billy Powell were here too! They had their truck and trailer parked in the driveway and their fifteen huskies and malamutes were each tied to a different fence post, separated so they couldn't fight. The dogs howled at night like wolves and barked incessantly in the daytime. Thankfully, we had no close neighbors or we could have been cited for disturbing the peace.

The Powells had a son, Billy, about Tino's age. Billy Jr., our Terri and the Zoppe kids added to the confusion with their shouting, running and playing.

Billy Sr. was a retired tight wire performer and after a few samples of our Kentucky bourbon climbed on the wire for the first time in years. Believe it or not, he was still a good wire walker. Billy's function in the act, besides being the family father, was to act as a groom and generally look after the animals and the equipment. Gee Gee, a blonde bombshell, was the star.

I often marveled at how strong her dogs seemed to be to pull her and the heavy sled, even though the sled was mounted on small wheels so it could be used inside. This day she offered to let me drive the dog team, so we hooked the dogs to the sled in our horse training ring and she showed me how to, "Gee and Haw them dogs," like she did. I did just as she said, and in the closed safety of my horse training track got the dogs started. Around that track I went! It was unbelievable how much power those five dogs generated. I was apprehensive and made some mistakes, so Gee Gee volunteered to show me how to drive them properly. I suggested she drive once around the track, then out the gate across the dam that formed the lake in our front yard and up the drive towards the house. I told her I would be at the top of the hill on the house side with the movie camera.

The plan sounded great and with a "hoot and holler," Gee Gee cracked the whip and shouted, "mush." The dogs took off, and what a show they put on. They flew around the track just as we had planned and then headed out the gate to the driveway. They were barking and running as fast as they could while Gee Gee, in all her blonde glory, was cracking her whip and shouting encouragement to the lead dog. They crossed the dam and started up the hill when suddenly one of the sled wheels hit a rock and jerked the lead dog off his stride and back over onto the number two dog in the team. All Hell broke loose and a dog fight like you never dreamed of was going full blast! Gee Gee was screaming, dogs were snarling and fighting. Jomar was a scene of absolute chaos! Billy Powell, Sr., who was standing with me as I took the movies, stood for a moment and sized up the situation. He switched his cigar to the other side of his mouth and very calmly, after getting to the scene of the battle, reached in and with sheer strength grabbed one of the big fighting dogs by the scruff of his neck and plucked him out of the fight like a tiny pup! Gee Gee grabbed that dog and Billy reached in for another one and in a matter of a very short time the fight was over. After a few choice cuss words Billy looked down and picked up a big canine tooth that one of his dogs had ripped out of another dog's mouth. I made some medical comment about that. He replied, "Hell, Doc, I'll wash it off and stick it back in the hole and it'll grow back in." As a veterinarian I was convinced it wouldn't work. And sure enough he did just that and sure enough it grew back!

It had been quite a day. We drove J.Y. and Martha back to the serenity of the circus and told Billy and Gee Gee to "tend the store" while we were gone. Everything had quieted down, and they went on about their business of feeding and caring for their animals.

That evening, not ten minutes after we came back home, a truck towing a house trailer turned into our driveway. We wondered who and what was next. It was Rudy Dockey and his boxer dogs. Just like this was an everyday occurrence, he slowed down and leaned out the window and in his broken German said, "Hello—I'm here, now we have something to get excited about." He never stopped but drove down the drive, across the dam and parked his outfit by the barn, making himself at home!

My clinic practice was not confined to just the local area. Some cases came from long distances. This made me feel good too, since my reputation had apparently reached far and wide. A phone call from Mr. Johnson in Punta Gorda, Florida, arranged an appointment to have an African leopard and a South American jaguar declawed. He brought the animals and left them two weeks in the clinic. At my insistence he had his shipping cages made to fit my squeeze chute and operating room space. When the three units were put together, it was a perfect fit. One thing to note about this case was that the jaguar and I got along fine. I could talk to him, and if I was careful stick my fingers through the bars of the cage and pet him. The leopard must have realized that I was the surgeon, though, and every time I went into the operating room where they were housed, all the fury of the jungle would break loose. I am certain, had that cat ever escaped and been loose in my clinic, I was a goner. She absolutely hated me. When Mr. Johnson came back to get his animals I told him about this and told him I would give him a demonstration of her dislike of me. The owner stayed in the kennel room and watched as I went into the surgery. The big spotted cat lunged, barred her long sharp teeth and roared. Even the walls shook! I came back out and Johnson laughed. He said, "Let's see what she does when I go in there." He opened the door, called the leopard by name and I'll swear, she purred like a house cat, lay down, rolled over and invited him to come pet her belly!

Other performers and their animals came through frequently. In fact, so frequently that the neighbors no longer stopped everything to see what was in the big trucks that so often pulled into the Martin Veterinary Clinic parking lot. Sometimes the neighborhood kids would stop in after school and ask if I had anything new or different.

I went to lunch one morning at a drug store lunch counter close to my office. When I came back there was a big tractor trailer rig parked in the street and this time there were quite a few people gathered around. I recognized them all as my neighbors and saw my friend Bucky Steele tending to eleven elephants all lined up in my front yard! He was on his way to Canada and needed, among other things, some health certificates. I fixed him right up and made friends with a new baby elephant that was the best broke punk I had ever seen. She made friends with the neighbors and let one of my technicians lead her around with the bull hook. Bucky soon was on his way and some months later wrote that the baby died after they got into Canada of some rare, exotic tropical disease. This poor creature no doubt had been sick for a long time.

An Englishman named John Radcliff was assigned to a Canadian government school in the Northwest Territory of Canada as a psychologist. His job was to be a guidance counselor to the Indians of the Yellow Knife area. One of the projects the school started was a singing group made up of five of the young Indian boys. John was in charge of this group and he thought they were talented enough to sing at a local fair as part of their schooling. They were so well received, and their singing so good, that it prompted other singing dates and eventually they migrated to the United States as a professional singing group. They became well known as the Chieftones. The boys soon had bookings at clubs, state and local fairs and exhibitions. As their reputation grew, so did their demand and they began making records. They were a successful and pleasing group of entertainers.

In their act they sang the song "Born Free" and at the very end of the song a full grown mountain lion, often called a cougar or puma, joined the group from her darkened cage. The lighting and the spectacular voices and the sudden appearance of this large cat made a tremendous impression on the audience. The presence of their beautiful animal became their trademark, but was soon a matter of concern with their agent and the people that engaged them that they might incur liability with this animal. It was decided to declaw the cat; that way they might avoid any liability. John Radcliff called me and we made the appointment to have the surgery done in my clinic.

Mary Helen and I invited them to park their bus at our house while they were in Ashland. They came the evening before the surgery was scheduled. We met all five—Jack, Jonas, Clifford, Vince and Richard—of these fine people and their manager, John Radcliff. They were polite, personable and easy to know. They introduced us to their big cat and with pride told us his name was Sim-Aw-Git. This meant "Chief" in their native language. Sim-Aw-Git was truly a fine specimen and more than being a prop in their act, in true Indian fashion, he was considered their brother.

The night before the surgery two of the boys, at Radcliff's insistence, removed all of the bedding from the large cage in the panel truck that housed the cat, and scrubbed it spotless with soap and water. Then they put in a deep bed of fresh straw for Chief's comfort after the operation. We scheduled the surgery for Sunday morning and took the cat to the clinic. We put him in the squeeze cage and I gave the anesthetic and removed the claws. It was a very clean, professional procedure and went without any problems. Slowly the cat started to wake up and when I thought it was safe to leave him, I suggested we drive back to our house and eat our dinner. Mary Helen had fixed a large beef roast and was prepared to serve it and a lot of ice cream for desert. Ice cream was the Indian boys' obsession. We all looked forward to our day.

At my suggestion to leave Chief in his cage where he was safe and cool, the boys held a quiet discussion and at once all five voted against my idea! There was no way that they were going to leave their lion alone in my hospital. I assured them their brother would be all right, but still they insisted they would take him home with them. After a lot of soul searching, and against my better judgement, I said OK. They carried their mountain lion brother out of my operating room and laid him in the back of the truck on the clean deep straw. At this stage the cat could sit up but was as yet unable to stand or walk. I was still apprehensive, but again I was overruled. It was warm in the truck and I didn't like that either. Again I suggested that the animal be left in the clinic. I even volunteered to stay with it myself. The vote was against me again and we drove the eight miles back to the farm. They parked the truck under the cooling shade of the oak trees in our yard.

The big cat seemed all right but I insisted that one of the Indian boys check on him at least every ten minutes. We waited for Mary Helen to finish fixing our meal and talked about many things including mountain lions, Indians, show business and their career. Every ten minutes one of the boys went to the truck to see if everything was OK. Vince made the last trip and looked in the truck door and turned and came running to the house to get me. Something had gone wrong.

I hurried out to the truck and found a very dead mountain lion, his head folded back under his body buried down under the deep straw! During the trip from the clinic to my house it was obvious that the heat of the vehicle and the deep straw resulted in the cat suffocating. I knew I had been right in objecting that we bring the recovering animal home so soon. I feel confident had we left him in my steel cage where it was cool and quiet, that cat would have recovered from the surgery with little or no problems. Of course I didn't dare tell them that.

Five Indians and their English boss and my wife cried. I felt like it but managed to hide my grief. Not a word was spoken for nearly two long hours. The boys were holding a wake for their departed brother! Finally, John Radcliff spoke directly to Jonas and said, "Jonas, it is time."

Without another word they got a shovel from the bus and walked out into our front yard to a spot where you could see off the hill and down into the valley. Jack, another one of the boys looked at me and pointed to a spot on the ground as if to ask— is it OK here? I assured them it was.

They buried their brother and when the last spade of dirt was put back, the grief was over. We went back and as hard as it was, they seemed to enjoy Mary Helen's dinner. Not another word was ever said about the lion. We remained friends for many years and Mary Helen and I followed them in their career. After a long time the group broke up. Radcliff went his way; the Indians went theirs. I learned a lesson that I never forgot, nor did I ever violate again. When it came to my patients, I made the decisions until I released them. That paid off many times in the following years.

Mary Helen and I planted a pink dogwood tree at the grave and every spring, when the tree blooms, we pay tribute to Sim-Aw-Git and think of his born-free spirit.

Never a day went by that I didn't get a phone call from some circus animal owner wanting my services or my advice. I never turned anyone down and I enjoyed every case and conversation I was involved in. I treated elephants with abscessed teeth, lions with broken toe-nails and chimpanzees with the sniffles. Lame horses, coughing and runny-nosed cats and elephants with the chills, flying trapeze artists and tumblers with aching backs and stilt walkers with sore legs all came my way! No two cases were ever alike.

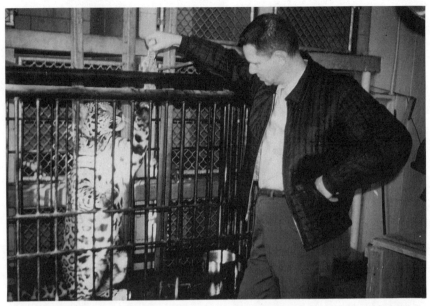

Dr. Martin got along very well with this South American jaguar prior to surgery, but its traveling mate, a leopard, was not friendly.

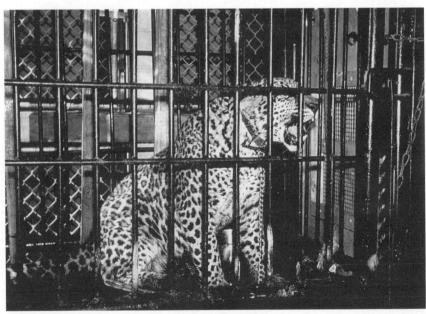

The African leopard belonged to Mr. Johnson and was very wary of Dr. Martin, who suspected that the cat remembered who the surgeon was.

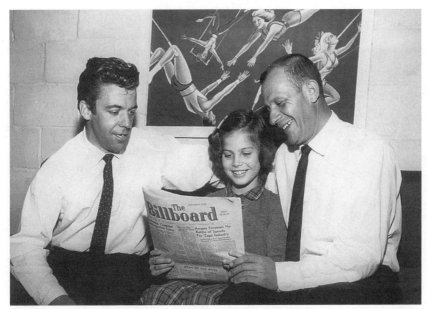

Terri Martin shows her real-life clown friends the story of her circus adventure in *The Billboard*.

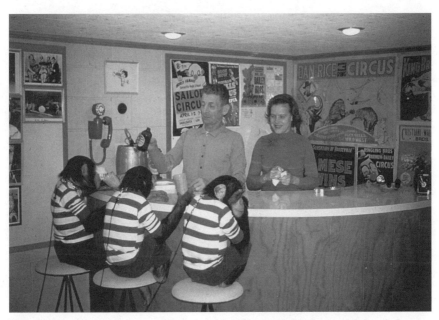

The Kirby Chimpanzees are served by Andrew Kirby and Mrs. Martin at Jomar, Dr. and Mrs. Martin's farm.

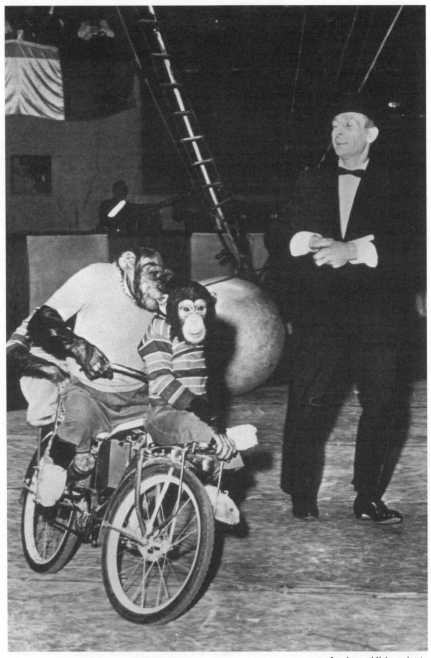

Andrew Kirby puts the Kirby Chimpanzees through their act.

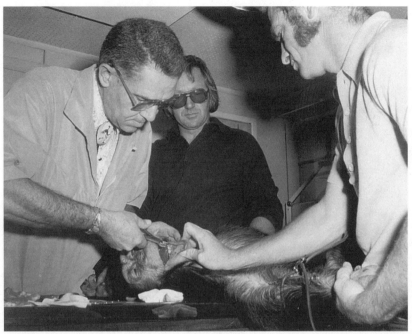

Dr. Martin, Frank Stephenson and clinic manager, Earl Hardin, extract an aching tooth from Stephenson's chimpanzee.

A Bengal tiger in the squeeze cage at the Martin Veterinary Clinic. This tiger had an infected tooth which made him very touchy! Tooth out—just another pussy cat?

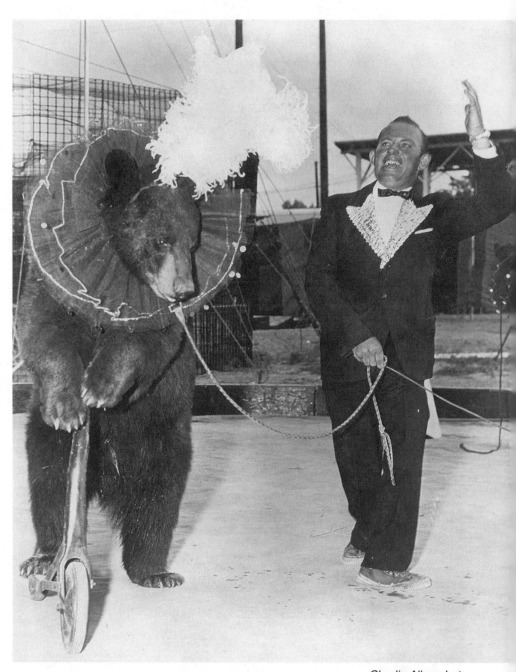

Charlie Allen was a wonderful animal "keeper" as is attested by this bear in prime condition.

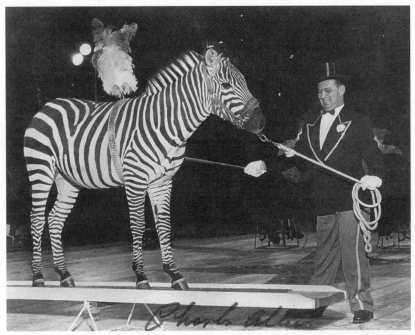

Charlie Allen and his football-kicking zebra. Without the bit, he was mean, mean, mean! Mr. Allen worked with the animals in the movie *Dr. Doolittle*.

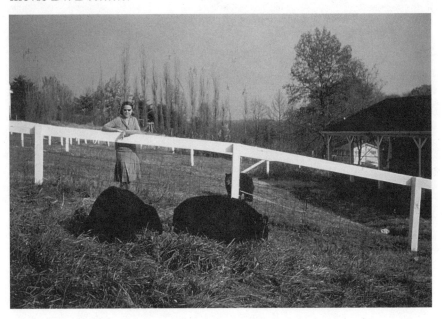

Mrs. Martin visiting Allen's bears in a paddock at the Martin Clinic who were chained together at the collar but could roam free. The small bear in the background was used in the TV series *Gentle Ben*.

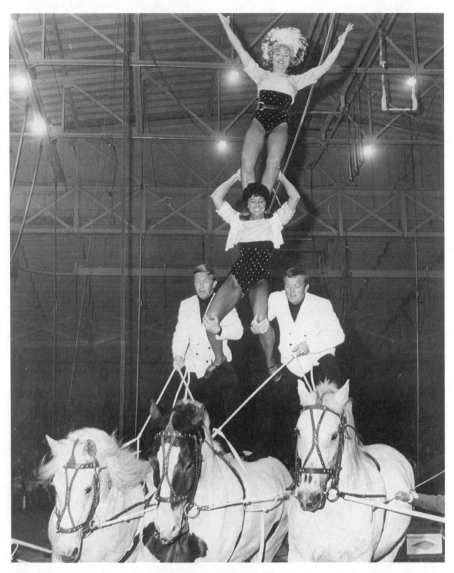

The Saxtons Riding Act was composed of three horses and the
Stephenson family bareback riders.

THE BIG SNAKE AND THE FORD FALCON

Late in the autumn of 1968, a friend from my wartime flying days sent me a newspaper clipping with a picture showing two farmers holding a dead snake. A note attached to the clipping asked if I remembered the snake that invaded my bamboo basha while we were flying in India. Of course I did and this note and the picture certainly did call back that incident. The snake described in the newspaper story was a python. It appeared to be about twelve or fifteen feet long. The newspaper article quoted one of the men as saying they found it coiled up in their garden and, "We shot it." I wrote my friend, thanked him for the clipping, and told him this story about an experience I had earlier with a big snake.

My reputation as a circus doctor was now pretty well established and it wasn't unusual to get called to address problems of the exotic animals.

Earlier that same summer, I received a phone call from a lady in Medora, Indiana. Her name was Silverlake. She and her family owned a small tent circus they were showing under the old Clark and Walters Circus title. The Silverlakes are one of my circus clients and they call me frequently when they have a sick circus critter. In this phone conversation, Mrs. Silverlake said they had three cases for me when I could make the show. She told me their elephant had a hook boil—an abscess—in its ear caused by over zealous use of an elephant hook. This was no big medical alert; I had treated several of these before. Case number two involved their chimpanzee who had the sniffles. This was not uncommon and unless the chimp was impossible to handle, it wasn't a major procedure. Case number three was the big one and she finally dropped the bomb when she told me her large python had not eaten for several months. "Would I please come as soon as possible and take care of them?"

Time, hard work and good fortune had improved my financial status and with this improvement I had the urge to fly airplanes again. Not only had I missed the excitement and fun of aviation, but now the practice covered such a large area, it could be a handy transportation tool. Through my reputation with the saddle horses and presence at the horse shows, I had recently acquired contracts to do the veterinary work on three horse farms in the Bluegrass area near Lexington. Lexington is one hundred and twenty five miles from my home in eastern Kentucky and before the airplane, it was a long hard day to drive to that part of the state, do my work and then get back home. It was often midnight when I finally made it back to Ashland. Acquisition of the airplane changed all of that. Instead of the two-hundred-fifty mile hard drive of five or six hours, I could make the round trip by plane in less than two hours.

I explained all of this to Mrs. Silverlake and then asked her for their route. After checking their itinerary, I told her I would be either in Clay City, Kentucky, or Morehead. Morehead had an airport and Clay City was served by a small airstrip in a little town close by. I told her since I would be flying, the exact place would depend on the weather. She understood. After she hung up, a slight shudder went through me at the mention of the word snake!

On the Clay City day, the weather was great. I dropped my medical bag in the backseat of my airplane and headed west into the mountain country. Clay City had no airport, but about seven miles up the scenic Kentucky Mountain Parkway was the little town of Stanton that proudly advertised a "3,500 feet, paved and lighted" airport. I found the field nestled in a little valley between mountains, landed and shut off the radios and the engine and looked around for an attendant. I couldn't find a soul but did see a small brick house nestled in the trees at the far end of the field. I walked to the building and knocked on the door.

My knock conjured up a nice little old lady—maybe eighty to eighty-five years old. I introduced myself and asked her if there was a taxi in the town. Her reply was direct and to the point, "Nope. Mister," she replied, "Ain't none. Where do ya want to go?"

I explained my mission and she told me her husband had a car and he would be glad to take me down the highway to the show town. I thanked her and waited while she rounded up her husband who, honestly, had to be at least ninety years old. He beckoned me towards a small shed and as I followed, I saw a Ford Falcon parked under the roof. The auto's vintage was unknown but it was obvious it had seen much younger and much better days. Both front fenders were dented and the rear bumper was wired on with some hay baling wire! I had no choice so I accepted the ride and we were off.

Back when I was a pilot in World War II, all of us had some frightening days when we flew our missions over war torn Burma and the mighty Himalayas Mountains we called the Hump. Believe me, the trip with the old man was far worse than the day back in December, 1944, when a Japanese fighter pilot tried to shoot me out of the sky! That day I didn't have time to be scared, or at least at the time— that came later.

This Ford Falcon adventure put the Zero day—for scariness— to shame. We roared down the expressway at full throttle, tires squealing with each turn as we careened from side to side around the graceful curves of the four-lane mountain road. Soon the exit ramp to the show town loomed ahead, and with another squeal of the tires, we turned off the ramp onto the main street of the little village. We never slowed down and drove straight through the town into the schoolhouse yard where the circus was set up. My driver slammed on the brakes, and finally the old Ford Falcon came to a stop in one hell of a cloud of dust! I climbed out of the car, gave the old man five dollars, and as if nothing unusual had happened, I thanked him for his services.

He smiled and never hesitated a bit when he said, "Sonny, do you want me to wait and take you back to the airport?"

Grateful to be alive, and not having enough nerve to ride with that old man again, I said, "No thanks, sir, one of my friends on the circus will take me back to my airplane." Our conversation was over. He turned the Ford around, gunned the motor, spun his wheels and left the circus lot in another cloud of summer dust.

Mrs. Silverlake and her son Mel saw me arrive and walked over to greet me. After shaking hands and saying the hellos, Mel asked me, "Have you had your lunch, Doc?" and without waiting for a reply added, "Let's go to the cook house and we'll get you something to eat."

I admitted I was hungry and, as we walked across the lot to the small cook house tent, I noticed everything was spotlessly clean—even the show kids, who by now had tagged behind us like rats after the Pied Piper! I smiled to myself, knowing my attendance was a special treat for these people. Had I not shown up at this town, the same gestures would be waiting for me at the next one! I ate my lunch and questioned my friends about the sick animals. I saved the snake discussion until last.

Question after question finally revealed that the snake had come from an exotic animal dealer up in Detroit. I was familiar with his operation and he did a good job. Mel Silverlake told me the snake had eaten pretty well for two or three months and then refused anything it was offered. It did have access to water and was really none the worse for wear. He told me they had tried everything from raw meat to live chickens. Mr. Snake refused his food. My next question was, "What did you feed him when you first got him?"

Mrs. Silverlake replied, "White rats."

About that time one of the kids who crowded around us held out a squirming guinea pig to look at and said, "Look, mister, what I got!"

I turned to Mel Silverlake and in a joking way asked him if they had ever tried feeding the snake a guinea pig.

Mel's mom exploded, "My God no, Doc, every kid on the show has one and if we did that I'd have a mutiny on my hands!"

I finished a good lunch and I decided I had put off my work long enough. Mel went to get his elephant so I could look at the hook boil. The show was set up in the local school yard and Mel walked the bull out into the middle of the baseball diamond for me to examine the sore ear. I couldn't reach the sore from where I stood so I asked Mel to lay her down. That worked, I cleaned and treated the wound—no problem. This didn't take long and before any mention could be made of anything else, my audience of school children, who had been let out for the day, and the local constable, applauded like I was a real hero! I accepted their applause. Then, before anyone could mention the word snake, I quickly said, "Let's go look at the chimp."

Chimps are a lot like kids when it comes to their illnesses but their temperament is completely different. They are extremely strong, generally mean and can hurt you in an instant. I never attempt to handle a chimpanzee, or any other circus animal for that matter, unless the trainer is there to control it. I am always extra careful when I treat or examine chimpanzees. They can grab and bite and inflict nasty wounds if you are careless. This guy was no problem. He was a well mannered monkey. I made my suggestions, told them I would leave some medicine and finally asked the inevitable question, "Where is the snake?"

You can see by this time that I am not a snake fan. You can also see I used every ploy in my book to escape treating that reptile, but sooner or later I had to face the facts that this obviously was the time.

With a nod of his head directed across the circus lot, Mel said, "Doc, its over in the back of that big truck."

We walked to the big truck. Up in the back was a large wooden box that had probably been used, before cardboard boxes came along, for shipping coffins. Mel whistled to some working men and told one of them to "get some help and come get this snake out, so the Doc can work on him."

Five men climbed up into the back of the truck. One man picked up a dirty old army blanket which was lying on the floor, and after very carefully opening the lid of the box, and making some remarks to his buddies, he tossed the blanket into the box and at the same time all five grabbed at the monstrous reptile. Twisting and squirming the snake soon appeared, the old army blanket over its head and all five men holding on for dear life. It was captured. Carefully they climbed down from the truck, each hugging his share of the heavy snake. Now it was my turn.

Once on the ground the men got a better hold and stretched him out for me to examine. I was just a little apprehensive, but I reached into my black medical bag and got my stethoscope. Carefully, I listened up and down the entire length of the snake—just like I knew what I was doing. I punched around and palpated different places and finally got up enough nerve to look at its head. I suddenly realized this monstrous reptile, a reticulated python, was truly a beautiful creature. The snake was at least fifteen feet long and looked just like the snake in the Ohio newspaper story. I went through further medical motions and mumbled a few low-toned, not understandable words under my breath—like doctors are sometimes supposed to do. I completed my extra lengthy examination and hanging my stethoscope around my neck I told the boss lady, who had been watching every move I made, I knew what was wrong with her snake. Then I added, "A shot will do the trick!" Fumbling around inside my little bag of medical magic I came up with the first bottle of medicine I touched. It was labeled "Sterile Saline Solution." I knew this wouldn't hurt my patient and I hastily filled a syringe. And then, very quickly, after using alcohol and a cotton swab, remarked for everyone to hear, "I'll give this shot in this old snake's hip and it won't be long 'till he's better." No one dared to ask where a snake had a hip.

My day's physical work was done and after dispensing some medicine for the chimp and elephant, I suggested when the circus came to a larger town, one that had a pet store, they buy some white rats. I further suggested they throw the old army blanket and a rat in the box with the snake. I added, "Don't open the lid for two days."

Mel drove me back to my airplane; paid his bill and we said our goodbyes. My last words to him were, "You, or your mother, call me in about a week, after you get the rats, and give me a report. It will take that long for the medicine to work." He promised me he would.

I hurried into my airplane and, without waiting to see if the little old man with the Ford Falcon was around, I taxied out and took off. I stayed low and headed down the road toward the circus lot where I put a good buzz job on the circus and the little town. The crowd at the circus looked up and waved. I rocked my wings, turned east, and headed home.

Ten days later, the phone rang and Mrs. Silverlake herself was quick to tell me, "Doc Martin, that shot you gave my snake in his hip has worked wonders. We got them rats like you told us and he's already ate six!"

I thanked her for the call and told her to never run out of white rats. I didn't tell her white rats were all that poor snake knew how to eat, since it had probably been born and raised in captivity, rats had been its total diet. I had that figured out before I ever made the trip to the circus.

I have, since then, wondered, after reading that newspaper story, if this could have been my old friend from the past that finally managed to get out of his coffin box only to be blasted by some frightened Ohio farmer. No one will ever know.

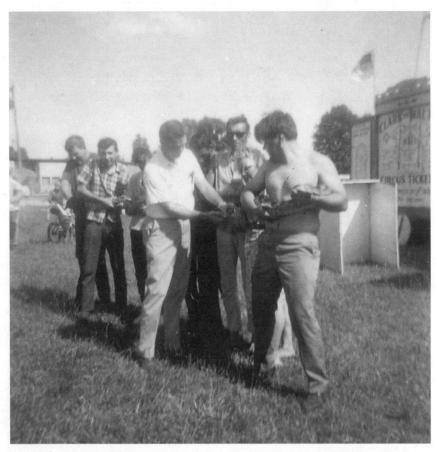

At the Clark & Walters Circus, Dr. Martin gave the fifteen-foot py-thon a shot in "his hip." After ten days and six fresh white rats, the snake was cured.

IT ISN'T ALL COTTON CANDY

In spite of the hoopla, spangles and cotton candy, mini-adventures with horses, itchy tigers, sick elephants, nasty camels, pigs and cows, the mainstay of my professional career had to be my small animal practice.

But personal implications, economics and a back injury that happened years earlier on Chris Crank's farm, made me make the decision to give up my large animal practice altogether. At first I left the stockyard with the intention of doing no more farm work. For a while I intended to continue caring for horses, but an old allergy seemed to accelerate and suddenly, every time I examined a horse, I would sneeze and sometimes develop a skin rash! My decision was made; I would restructure my practice, and the Martin Veterinary Clinic would become a small animal facility. I did retain my circus animal practice.

A typical day could be often more fun, and sometimes more exciting, than the circus! Over the course of time, I saw sick dogs, sick cats, pet birds, gerbils, ferrets and snakes and any other kind of animal you could make a pet of. Most patients, of course, were cats and dogs and their problems were, as a general rule, routine. There were some exceptions. I am sure many of these were generated by my circus background.

In the mornings office hours were from ten until noon. We took a lunch break and then resumed scheduled hours from two o'clock until five. Those were the published hours, but it was seldom I got home before six or seven in the evening. Then, later on most nights, I would go back to the clinic to medicate or check on a patient. Once in a while, after the office was closed for the day, I made house calls.

I was late getting to the office one morning and there were already people in the waiting room. I put on my white office coat, stepped into the waiting room and asked, "Who's first?"

"I am, Doc. My—" the client mumbled something I didn't hear, "is in the car." He hurried out toward his car and I turned around and walked into one of the examination rooms. In a matter of a minute or two, the client, a young man about twenty-five years old, said, "Here he is, Doc, see what's wrong with him."

I looked at this fellow and I was looking at a person who already was trying my patience. Something about him and his pet just didn't click. "Well, sir, just put him up here on the table and tell me about him."

The man, with a little snicker, said, "You put him up there."

I hesitated a minute knowing this man had something on his mind about me, or his pet, or both. I used my usual ploy when I got in a situation where the owner wouldn't put his or her animal on the table and said, "I can't lift that big dog—I have a very brittle back. You are big and strong and after all, he is your dog."

The owner looked down at his pet and finally reached down and very carefully picked him up and put him on the table. This was a dog—of some sort. There was just a feeling that it wasn't an ordinary dog. He had short hair, weighed about forty pounds and there was something about his head and the shape of his mouth that I wasn't familiar with. After giving him a quick look over, but never putting my hands on him, I asked my client, "Just what have you brought to me?" I continued, "This is not an ordinary dog and I don't think you are being fair to me by not telling me what you are up to." By this time I was getting pretty disturbed.

"Hell, Doc,"—already he was too familiar—the term "Doc" is reserved for use by my friends and those who use it reverently. This person was neither—he wasn't my friend and there certainly was no reverence. "I didn't really think you knew what he was." He looked at me and finally said, "It's an Australian dingo. I had him shipped in here—and I call him Aussie." He gave me that defiant look again and said, "You learned something this morning, didn't you?"

I was now about ready to lose what serenity I had, but I cooled down and calmly read him the riot act about bringing a potentially dangerous animal in like he did. I added his dingo could have hurt someone and also told him that I felt he was not one damned bit smart for acting with me like he did.

"My Gawd, Doc," Again he did it! "I meant no harm."

I was in command now and very carefully I examined this interesting animal and got its history. This Australian visitor dog kept licking his mouth like he had a sore throat. Carefully I took his temperature. He had three degrees of fever. I asked the owner if he could open his pet's mouth, "Real wide, I want to look down his throat."

The dingo owner paused, and after a second or two, he said, "Well, I don't know."

Before he could say anything else, I said, "Do it." Very carefully he did and sure enough there were two great big inflamed tonsils. And sure enough, this animal's mouth wasn't at all like most dogs. The molars were wider and were set in a massive lower jaw bone. There were also more molars than in the domestic dog. All of this was designed for killing and crushing bone. I took my time looking at this arrangement of dental tools and decided I had made a good judgement call when I refused to pick up Mr. Dingo. I gave this first cousin to our dog an injection of penicillin and dispensed some tablets to help fight the infection. It also went through my mind that he might get bit in the process of giving the pills. I was determined to get even with this guy.

"Bring him back in the morning but be sure there isn't anyone in the waiting room before you bring him in."

"Doctor Martin," now, showing me a little respect, "I am sorry if I upset you, but I knew you had a lot of experience with wild animals. I know you are a veterinarian for most of the circuses and I thought it would be old stuff to you."

The next morning he was back. He picked the dingo up and put him on the table without my asking and told me his pet was much better. He paid his bill and thanked me again. I took care of that strange canine for two years, giving him his shots and tending his regular needs. In all that time, this man never again addressed me as "Doc," never again tried to fool me and we developed a good client-doctor relationship. Eventually the dingo just disappeared—maybe he died or maybe the owner moved to another town. If he did move someplace else, I hope the next veterinarian realizes that that Aussie is not an ordinary dog.

My ordinary day began with the technician presenting me with all of the patient charts, and one by one we would examine the animals and medicate them or make decisions to discharge them. After visiting with every animal, we set up the surgery schedule for the day. The usual day's surgery included one or more ear-cropping operations —a procedure I was particularly adept at, spays and castrations and the routine minor surgeries. Dystocia in dogs and cats was challenging just like it was in the large animals. Frequently we resorted to cesarean sections. Fracture repair was an everyday occurrence, and most of the broken bones were repaired with bone pins, wires, nuts and bolts and bone plates. I became quite proficient at animal orthopedics. After surgery was done, I conducted my office hours and saw new patients. It was an interesting day; no two spays or neuters were ever alike, nor were any two fracture cases the same. Veterinary internal medicine was truly fascinating. We saw all of the pathology you see in human medicine and some just indigenous to animals. I mentioned one time to a lady pathologist that pathology was pathology whether it was human or animal. She sneered and denied my statement. She showed her lack of respect for my profession and her lack of knowledge about overall medicine. Maybe she was just jealous because most veterinarians command so much respect from the general public. Today a lot of MDs don't.

The very nature of animal medicine caused us to see a variety of clinical cases. Trauma cases, parasite problems, and skin cases are very common. We also encountered many seasonal and environmentally related sickness—for an example, animals poisoned on antifreeze during the winter months. Our infectious diseases such as canine distemper, hepatitis, leptospirosis, or rabies, were easy to control with the refined vaccines that were available

When I finally developed my diagnostic laboratory, the pattern changed. The technician would do the blood work or laboratory tests I ordered. I would make the examination and determine what to do, then order the proper treatment. The technician and our lay help did the actual medicating, and I followed the progress from day to day until the case was dismissed. I did all of the immunizations myself. No technician ever gave a vaccine unless I was there to supervise it. This policy prevented any liability, or client denial about a pet's having been given the vaccine if something went wrong.

The business part of small animal medicine and the changing times required several hours a day of uninteresting but necessary office work. There were records to update, bills to pay and meetings to attend. When I wasn't doing some of these things, I was reading about some new technique or procedure just developed.

In spite of all the precautionary measures and careful planning, humans make mistakes. A lady from southern Ohio brought us a beautiful Scotch collie dog. She admitted him into the hospital and told us she would leave him for ten days. "While he is here," she asked me, "Would you mind fixing him?" I questioned her and she assured me that she did indeed want him castrated. She made a grimace and looking at her dog said, "He's so nasty at times!"

Two days later I put a big, good looking male collie on my operating room table and did the requested surgery. No problems or complications.

Eight days later my lady client came after her collie and took him home. About an hour after she left, she called and very firmly let me know I had cheated her. Indignantly she said to me, "You never touched my dog!" I told her something had gone wrong and I would call her right back. I hoped she was an understanding person.

I had a meeting with Earl and the office girls, and we checked our records. We had indeed castrated a male collie eight days earlier. Further search of the records revealed that there were two large male Scotch collies in the clinic at the same time. An absolutely horrible realization hit me—I had castrated the wrong dog!

I had to face reality, no matter what the consequences were, and I called the owner of the castrated dog. I just knew I was about to own the most expensive collie in the world! A man answered my phone call and before I could say anything, he thanked me for operating on his dog. I had forgotten about a year earlier we had discussed doing this and I had put it off several times because I was out on a circus or some other trip. I sat by my phone in dumbfounded shock. My man said, "Doc, just send me the surgery bill along with the board bill." He added, "I just knew I could always depend on you and your work!"

As soon as I hung up, I called the lady in Ohio and told her some story to ease her down and apologized for any inconvenience she might have had. I asked her to bring her dog back and I would do the work for her. Later in the week she returned and I did castrate the right dog this time. That case was closed, but I came about an inch from getting into some real trouble.

About a week later a young girl brought in her mother's red cocker spaniel to have her spayed. As I walked through the kennel to the surgery room, I noticed two red cockers caged side by side. Both wagged their tales at me. I stopped dead in my tracks and called the technician and asked her which dog I was to spay. She said, "Doctor, the red one of course."

I showed her two "red ones" and got on the phone and had one of the owners come identify his dog. I could never in the world have made the same mistake twice and gotten away with it. I spayed the correct dog but that same day, in less than an hour after this happened, I ordered some name collars. From that day on, every animal we admitted to the clinic was tagged with a special ID collar with the owner's name on it as well as what the animal was in the clinic for. That solved the problem.

Chinchillas were in vogue. I got my share of that business. It was get rich for some and a go-broke for others. I got to the office early one morning and was surprised to see my neighbor, Benton, waiting for me. He was in the chinchilla business, and I had been to his house out of curiosity to see his operation. It was interesting and a new experience, and from what I could see, Benton was doing a good job. I asked him, "What can I do for you this morning?"

"Doc," he was entitled to use this term—he was a friend, "This female is having trouble having her babies." I examined her and found no evidence of a normal birth even though the little animal was in hard labor.

"Benton, I think we are going to have to do a C-section. Maybe we can save the babies—at least the chance of saving the mother is very good."

"Can I watch you do the surgery?" he asked, and I told him it would be OK—if the mother didn't object! He appreciated my joke.

I anesthetized the little animal and the surgery was routine until I delivered the first baby. I ordinarily used a metal basket, lined with a turkish towel, to hold my c-section deliveries while I was operating. I delivered the first little one. It was about one inch long and an absolute live wire of activity. Stormy put the baby in our basket and turned to help me with the second one when Benton piped up in a startled voice, "Doc, that darned baby is running away!" Sure enough the newly delivered, still dripping wet, little baby was running around like an adult creature. It was out of the basket and on the table, its little legs flying and zigzagging all over the surgical drapes! Benton caught it and held it while I delivered another and finished the surgery. Two new chinchillas were in our world and I had saved the mother. These were the only newborn creatures I ever saw that were completely able to walk and run as soon as they came into our world. I did two more of these operations before the fad faded away, and you can bet I had made arrangements to confine the babies as soon as they were delivered.

SOME THINGS WERE BIZARRE, SOME UNUSUAL, SOME PURE BUSINESS

Not all of my entertainment or excitement came from the Big Top experiences. Not all circus veterinary medicine was a big adventure. Only on occasion was it different.

My clinic practice was no different. In a veterinary practice such as the one I had created, most of the incidents were usually just plain business deals. They lacked the glamour most people imagined went on behind my clinic doors. But on the other hand, like the circus work, some were unusual and on occasion they were bizarre.

At the beginning of this writing, I told about the day I was stuck in the snowstorm and after trudging nearly a half mile through the deep snow to his house, had my friend, Lace Hardin, get his mules and pull my car out of the snow drift. Lace insisted that I go to his barn and examine his two three-year-old stallions that were not even halter broke. They were vicious like some of the wild animals I treated in my circus practice. I asked him at the time how he was going to manage to break them. His answer was, "Doc Martin, they won't be no trouble to break—after you geld 'em, come this spring."

As I drove back home that night, I recalled my busy day and what it had produced. A lot of things went through my mind but I gave second thoughts to those two mean horses and Mr. Hardin's remarks about gelding his stallions, ". . . come next spring." Now this was a matter of business and after the snows melted, sure to his word Lace Hardin called on a warm May day and asked me to come and, ". . . cut them colts."

I made the appointment and told him to be sure we had at least two men to help us. He agreed to that.

On the appointed day, exactly at my appointed time, I drove into the barnyard of the Hardin farm. Lace was waiting for me. He had two other men there to help. They had been drinking whiskey and one of them offered me a drink. I told him, "No, but thanks anyway." Then I asked, "Where are the horses?"

One of Lace's hired men spoke up and said, "Them horses is out in the field. We didn't think you'd be here so soon." Had it not been for my good Hardin family relationship, and remembering that awfully cold day when Lace and his mules pulled me through the snow and mud, I would have turned around and gone back home.

About this time Mrs. Hardin showed up. I could see that she was angry and with steel in her voice and fire in her eyes, she demanded that all three of them get to the field and get the horses in the barn. She apologized to me and invited me in for a glass of cold milk. We went to the kitchen and had a nice talk while we both recovered our tempers.

Her orders were promptly attended to, and before long here came the three men herding the two big stallions toward the barn and only from habit, because they were always fed there, did they go into their individual stalls.

After close to four months of wondering how I was going to handle these wild horses, I finally had a plan. First I had to catch one, and somehow get a needle into his jugular vein, and give him a big dose of chloral hydrate solution, which would put him sound asleep. If I got lucky enough to do that, I could castrate those studs. Carefully opening the stall door, I managed to throw my lasso rope around one horse's head and then snubbed my rope to a post in the barn wall. All hell broke loose. If you ever saw a mad wild animal it was this horse. He kicked and reared and squealed and lunged and fought everything in the stall, real and imaginary! I thanked my Maker we were outside in the safety of the aisle of the barn. Following my instructions, my helpers tightened the rope every time the horse lunged, eventually drawing him up tight to the post. The tight rope around his neck shut off his wind and he sank unconscious to the floor. In a flash I had the needle in the jugular, loosened the lasso so he could breathe and sighed in relief as I saw this mighty horse relax from my medicine. I finished tying him up and did the simple operation. Lace and his two helpers, against my better judgement, toasted my success with another drink from their whiskey bottle. When that horse recovered enough to be safe to leave alone, I lassoed the other one, choked him down, put him to sleep with the chloral hydrate, and castrated him. The job I had been so concerned about ever since the big snowstorm was over. It had been rewarding. Besides getting my car pulled out of the mud and snow, I got paid hard cash for a risky job. I also gained a fortune in satisfaction for what I had done. On my way out of the barn I stopped by the mule stalls and said hello to long eared Sam and patted old Barney on the nose. Now I consider this case as strictly business.

Just before bedtime one night, the phone rang and a lady on the line asked, "Doctor Martin, would you make a house call? I know its late but our little dog is having some sort of a spell—its almost like a seizure." She went on to say, "She has been so well and, oh yes if it means anything, she just had a litter of puppies four days ago."

That remark got my attention and I realized that this mother dog had eclampsia, a disease that is very similar to milk fever in cows. It is basically a mineral imbalance that sometimes comes with birthings and if unattended, can be fatal. I asked for directions to her house and told her I would be there in a few minutes.

"Thank you so much. Come downtown to the Freedom Hotel and come through the middle door and up to the second floor. My apartment is the last one down the hall."

Now this hotel was old. It had seen better days and had been closed as a hotel for several years. Its history dated back to the nineteen twenties. The building was a good candidate for replacement. I knew nothing about it other than it was there.

I drove into town and parked in front of the hotel. I checked my medical bag for what I thought I would need and after locking my car, went into the building. I climbed the wooden steps to the second floor. At the landing I looked down the hall toward the end where my client said she lived and I got the surprise of my life. There were three doors on each side of the hall and one door, obviously the client's, was at the end. Standing in each door watching my arrival was a young woman. These girls were fairly pretty and I was quick to notice that each one was dressed in a house coat—and apparently that was all!

I addressed the first girl and asked, "The lady with the sick dog?" She pointed a finger down the hall.

I knocked. A very polite older woman answered and at once thanked me for coming. I treated the dog which did indeed have eclampsia. I finished and very graciously accepted a cup of coffee and collected my fee. She promised to call me early the next day and report on mother dog and puppies. She thanked me again and I left. Every one of the girls in that place thanked me as I went by their rooms.

I had heard about red light districts and houses of prostitution and had seen some during the war but this was my first personal experience with one. All my male friends for the next few weeks jokingly asked me how I got paid! I was fast to answer, "With cash!" Not every case was so—let's say, bizarre.

Some cases were unusual and not every unusual case involved the animal. Instead, the owner made it interesting. One afternoon during office hours, a young woman and her six-year-old son came to pick up a dog I had been treating. While I was talking to her about the dog and its after-care, her little boy was as busy as could be opening all of the cabinet doors and pulling things out. I looked at the mother and then glared at the boy and neither responded. I just shut each door as he opened them. Finally I could take no more and in a very nice quiet way, I asked the lady to please control her child. She absolutely ignored me. About two more cabinet doors and then he found a box of examination gloves and started to pull them out of the box and put one on his little hand.

"Lady, control your kid—please!" After saying this I turned to the child and said directly to him, "If you belonged to me, I'd bust your bottom."

The mother still said not another word and about that time the little devil took a big leap and hit me just above the knees with both feet and yelled, "Kungfoo!" I was a victim of the martial arts by a six-year-old karate expert!

Hart, one of my technicians, came through the door from the kennel with the lady's dog on a leash, not realizing what I had just gone through. I was standing there in a state of shock and utter surprise that a grown woman would allow her child to get so out of hand. The woman snatched the leash from Hart and said to her child, "Let's get out of this mean man's place." I glared after them. If looks could have killed, that lady and her nasty little kid would have been dead.

She stopped just before leaving the examination room and asked me, "How much is my bill?" I made a quick calculation, doubled the price just to satisfy my hurt ego and thanked her for her business. I never saw her—or that brat again.

Politics never was my forte. I knew some elected officials, but never used them for any personal gain. Most of my experience with them involved proposed leash laws, rabies control programs or situations of that nature.

In the very early days of my practice, while I was still doing farm work, I was called to a farm in Carter County—the county west of where we lived—to look at a sick cow. This farm was about thirty-five miles from my office and was off the main roads back in the hill country. I finished my work and the owner and I walked toward my car, enjoying a brief conversation. As we stood there an older man carrying a walking stick came slowly walking down the dusty country road and said hello to us.

My client, who was busy writing me a check, looked up and said, "Well hello, gov'nor, what you doing in this part of the county?"

The old man said, "I've been over to Mr. Tabor's for a visit. My nephew brought me out here." He turned and started toward the house. "I'll go say hello to your missus while you two are doin' your business."

I must have sensed something because I asked my client why he called this man, "Governor"?

"Doctor, that's Mr. Fields—used to be gov'nor of Kentucky. He's a nice old gentleman and visits around when he can."

The governor came back from his short visit with the lady of the house and my client introduced me to him. We shook hands and he asked, "Doctor, will you give me a ride into Grayson?" Grayson was the county seat and I had to go through there to get back home.

"Yes, sir. I would be more than pleased to take you to town." We both said our goodbyes and Governor Fields and I had a very nice visit. We talked about my work and I asked him about his days in politics. He wanted to know if I was politically inclined and I told him no—I was too busy in the veterinary business. In the course of our conversation, I commented the only political aspiration I ever had was to be a Kentucky Colonel. Governor Fields chuckled and re-marked, "I bet I signed thousands of those certificates." Before long we got to Grayson and I let the governor out in front of the county courthouse. Today there is a bronze statue in that courthouse yard of Governor William Jason Fields, Governor of the Commonwealth of Kentucky, 1923-1927.

A few years later another governor did indeed honor me with a commission as a Kentucky Colonel.

A year or so after this chance meeting with the governor, I had an occasion to treat a cow with milk fever almost in sight of the governor's home in Pleasant Valley—a small community in Carter County a few miles west of the county seat. I don't remember who owned the cow but on the phone the farmer told me to "come to the cemetery just after you pass the Fields' home." I told the man I knew exactly where that was. He said, "I'll meet you there—the cow is at the top of the hill next to the grave yard fence. Come to the gate at the west end of the cemetery."

It was a pretty, warm summer day and I asked Harry Steele, my neighbor across the street, if he wanted to go with me on the call. Most people liked to travel with me as they never knew what was going to happen next. Harry asked if this was an exciting case and I said, "No—just an old cow down with milk fever."

We talked and had a nice visit as I drove the nearly forty miles to Pleasant Valley. We passed Governor Fields' boyhood home and I told Harry the story about my meeting the governor. Just a few hundred yards past the Fields' house was the cemetery and sure enough, the cow's owner was waiting for us at the gate to his pasture.

He thanked me for coming and after I introduced him to Harry, he said, "Doctor, the cow has drug herself through the fence and she's in the cemetery." We walked on up the hill and there she was stretched out like she was dead. Flies were walking across her eyeballs and the only indication that she was alive was an occasional shallow breath. I checked her heart and started the medicine into her jugular vein.

I had no sooner started the treatment when, down at the main gate in the graveyard, a hearse pulled up and the driver got out. I noticed him look up the hill where Harry and the farmer and I were doctoring this cow. He was the undertaker. He walked up the hill to us and introduced himself and wanted to know if we could help him.

He said, "If you gentlemen wouldn't mind, I need your help to be pallbearers. There's just me and the preacher and two old ladies here." He hesitated and then said, "Them that promised to be here didn't show up!" His voice rang with Kentucky twang and after the absolute surprise of being asked to participate in a funeral, I told him I was willing but he would have to wait until I treated the cow. He said, "I thank ya'. When you're ready just come to the hearse."

We finished treating the cow and once she started to respond, I took my lariat and fashioned a halter with it and tied the cow to a big heavy tombstone. Then we walked down the hill and helped carry the casket up to a freshly dug grave not far from where my patient was now blinking her eyes and coming back to life.

I did have the decency to take off my dirt covered coveralls and the three of us, the two old ladies, the preacher and the undertaker bowed our heads in respect to the dead.

After it was all over and we were back in my car on the way home,

Harry Steele spoke up and remarked, "Jack, I thought you said this would just be an ordinary milk fever case."

I laughed and commented that you never knew what to expect if you were a hillbilly veterinarian.

SOME THINGS PURE BUSINESS—
BUT STRANGE

The telephone is the life blood of most businesses and mine was no different. After a very busy morning when the phone never seemed to stop ringing, worked in between the "how much" calls and the "I would like to make an appointment" ring-ups, I had a call from the Ashland Chief of Police.

"Doctor, this is Chief Howard. We have some items down here at the hospital and I wonder if you would have time to come down and look at them for us? Just come when it is convenient."

That's all the chief told me over the phone, and of course I was as curious as I could be about such a strange request. It was close to noon and I told Stormy that I might as well go down there during our lunch break.

I arrived at the hospital, and no sooner had I walked in the door when a Kentucky State Police Officer, who was obviously waiting for me, motioned for me to follow him down the hall. As I turned the corner to follow this man, I suddenly realized that there were several other officers there. The law was represented by Chief Howard, the county sheriff and two of his deputies and three more state police officers! There were also two lawyers from the county attorney's office and Dr. Stewart, the head pathologist from our hospital. Something unusual was in the making.

The Chief of Police filled me in on the story. On a routine patrol by one of his officers to the city dump, the policeman saw what appeared to be some arms or legs on the pile of trash. He called his boss, Chief Howard called the coroner and then he called me.

As we walked down the hall toward the pathology section I asked

Dr. Stewart, my pathologist friend, if by chance they had taken any X-ray photographs of these limbs. He said, "Yes, that's the very first thing I did. Let's step in here and take a look at the films." We turned into the X-ray department and there on the Picker Viewer were four X-ray films of these specimens.

I studied the films for a moment and it dawned on me why I had been called. The police could not identify these limbs and it was up to me to decide if they came from a human or some other being. One look and then it was my turn to light up my halo. I saw that these dismembered arms or legs had no indication of having a thumb. This meant they were not primates, which ruled out the possibility that they were of human origin. The films also revealed an unusually long bone in the leg specimens that was like the bone in a human's heel. I commented on the extreme length of these bones and again suggested they were different from homo sapiens. I explained this to everyone and there was a very audible sound of relief. The next question was, what were they, where did they come from?

We left the X-ray department and walked on down the hall to the hospital morgue. An attendant went into the large cooler and brought out two big plastic bags with the arms and legs in them and put them on their autopsy table. These dismembered limbs had no skin on them nor did they have any fingernails. The tissue was not decomposed and showed no sign of any trauma other than they had been skinned. It also was evident these specimens involved two animals—one quite a bit larger than the other. There were two arms and two legs from each individual. The pathologist handed me a pair of postmortem gloves, and after I put them on, I took these gruesome objects out of their bags and tried to identify them. In the bottom of one of the bags were several strands of black hair perhaps two or three inches long.

After considerable thinking, I finally suggested these body parts came from two bears. One of the officers queried why there were no nails. I thought again and offered that they had been saved when the skin was removed for a trophy! By this time I was an absolute celebrity—well justified to wear my big smile. Investigation later revealed that bear hunting season was open in West Virginia and some other states but we never found out where these came from. Perhaps they had been killed illegally and the hunter figured the city dump as the best place to dispose of the leftover parts. I felt good about this case since I considered it a public service as well as a learning experience for me.

Sometimes good things happen to you. Sometimes it was the other way around. Here is an example of how close you can come to getting into big trouble and come out smelling like a rose when it was all over. This stud horse story came pretty close to ending my career or at least getting me into a legal bind.

One evening one of my horse clients called me up and wanted to know if I could castrate his horse for him. He said, "Doc, can you do it tomorrow—the sign's right!" My client, like so many of my Kentucky friends, did nothing until the Zodiac sign was in the correct position! "If you can," he continued, "I'll put him in your clinic barn before I go to work in the morning. You know which stud I'm talkin' about, it's the palomino."

I told him, "Sure I'll do it. You come back and get him tomorrow after supper." The deal was done.

Dr. Henderson, my circus veterinary friend, was visiting me that week and we had often discussed my standing castration procedure. Up until this time, he had never seen it done. Now we had the opportunity—we had a stud to work on. Henderson went with me the next morning on two farm calls. We talked about the horse operation, the technique and its advantages over the complete anesthetic, laid-down-tied-up procedure. He was eager to watch.

Before we got back to the clinic we stopped at a little restaurant and ate some soup beans and corn bread for lunch—one of J.Y.'s treats when he visited us. When we got to the office, Earl, my helper, had the instruments sterilized and all was ready. I told Earl to go down to the barn and get the palomino and we would do the surgery up at the main building.

Henderson and I waited and he commented on what a good looking stud Earl was leading up the hill from the barn. I knew the horse from some previous work, and as I got my instruments ready I grunted an approval. We were standing at the side of the clinic next to the parking lot, and I suggested to Dr. Henderson that we get on with it to avoid any embarrassment if the neighbors or some client would come in while I was operating. I did make one comment, "My client has done something good for this colt. He looks like a different horse from the last time I saw him."

Earl put the horse's head in a corner and put the twitch on the palomino's nose. I tied the rope in his tail and fastened it up over the framework of some steel dog runways.

I got my knife and was just ready to make the first bold incision into the scrotum when a man shouted out, "What in the hell are you going to do to my horse?" I straightened up and knew right away I didn't have the right animal! How close had I come to making a really big mistake by operating on the wrong horse?

Now I knew whose horse it was and I faked a laugh and said, "Bill, we saw you walking up the street and we thought we would play a little joke on you—it sure worked out fine, didn't it?" My lie worked. He believed the story. He made a remark that he didn't think my humor was too funny.

Henderson was absolutely amazed, I was darn near in a state of shock and of course Earl had no idea of what was going on. Bill told me he had put his horse in the barn next "to another yellow horse" just before lunch. He wanted me to worm it. Well, I wormed Bill's stud. I made some more remarks about the joke we played on him. After he was gone, Earl went to the barn and got the right "yellow horse."

For years after that episode, when I mentioned castrating a horse to Dr. Henderson, he would always comment, "Just be sure you have the right one, Jackson." I consider that case in the unusual category!

Ernest Baker's bloated cows were another one of the unusual cases that comes to my mind.

It was early spring and the usual early rains had most of the creeks out of their banks and some of our sections isolated by flood waters. Ernest called me one afternoon and told me that his entire dairy herd of Holsteins were forced into his alfalfa field by the high water and they were all bloated—bad! "Doc, you can't get here, all of the roads are flooded. What can I do? I'm in a hell of a shape."

I had done a lot of work at his dairy and had on occasion passed a stomach tube down some of his cows. I said, "Ernest, take a piece of garden hose and see if you can pass a tube into their stomachs like I do. That should let the air out." While I was telling him this, I was scrambling through my mind trying to figure out what I could do over the phone that might save his herd.

"Doc, I tried that hose trick already and all I get is foam!"

Right there I knew his cows had frothy bloat and that was sometimes hard to handle. The best cure was to relieve the surface tension of the stomach contents and get the animals out of the source of trouble. I didn't know how he was going to get his cows moved, but I thought I knew how to cure his problem. I asked, "Ernest, does your wife have any Tide washing detergent powders?"

"Hold on a minute, Doc, I'll ask her." There was silence for a moment and then he came back on the phone and said, "She sure does, as a matter of fact, she said she picked up a new giant sized box last week at the grocery store. What's that got to do with my sick cows?"

I explained to him that frothy bloat was not one pocket of stomach gas like most simple bloat cases, but instead, was caused by thousands of tiny bubbles resulting from the fermenting wet alfalfa the cattle had eaten. The detergent would decrease the surface tension of the stomach contents and that would cause the bubbles to burst. I assured him it wouldn't hurt the cows and in view of the fact that I couldn't get there, it might save the herd. I told him to start right away and to call me back every hour or so and report on their condition.

In about an hour the phone rang. It was Ernest reporting. "Doc, by gosh it worked. Every one of my cows are better!"

I tucked that information away in my head and used it several times when I had a bloated cow.

Some things were just routine veterinary medicine, even though they seemed strange. This case is just one of those, albeit it had a "Vanbibber" twist to it.

One night my insurance salesman friend Charles called me to his dairy to look at a newborn calf. The calf was stretched out, almost lifeless, pale and looked to be near death. It was a victim of what I called Baby Calf Syndrome. Someplace in its birthing the chemistry didn't function just right and the newborn was almost in a state of shock. Unless attended to promptly, these animals died. I had unusually good luck by giving these calves a blood transfusion with blood from their mothers.

When I got to the dairy one of Charles' friends, Amos Vanbibber, was there. He was usually a likeable person, but at times quite cynical. He looked at me and then over at the sick calf and told Charles he was wasting his time fooling with me. Amos turned and walked out of the barn into the dark towards his house which was about one hundred yards away.

I fixed up my transfusion equipment and proceeded to draw a pint of blood from the mother cow getting ready to infuse it into the calf. I had no sooner filled the pint bottle when Amos, his curiosity fully aroused, came back into the barn.

He stood there and again expressed his doubt about Charles using good judgement to treat a dead calf. I ignored his remarks and Charles did, too.

Charles held the baby still and I inserted the needle into its jugular vein and started the life saving blood on its way. Slowly I let it drip and it seemed like with every drop the calf got better. It was blinking its eyes and even attempted once to get on its feet. Charles and I knew we were winning. Amos wasn't yet ready to admit we were right.

Finally I emptied the bottle and withdrew the needle. The baby calf was obviously much better. I waited around for a while and pretty soon we helped the calf get on its feet.

Amos didn't know what to say and finally sputtering something we didn't understand, walked out into the night and back home. He never mentioned that calf again to me but Charles tells me Amos told everyone in the neighborhood what a good job I had done.

Now Amos Vanbibber at times had a doubting personality, but he wasn't a belligerent person, and he never was rude or deliberately defiant. Over the years, though, I saw some that did defy you and even made it an issue to try and intimidate.

In the mid 1960s, most doctors held evening office hours. I was no exception. Mine were from six-thirty until eight, or whenever I saw the last patient.

One evening when my office hours were to start, a car careened into the parking lot and stopped with a jolt. The car's wheels had no sooner stopped turning when a very excited woman got out of the car and ran into my waiting room.

"Doctor," she shouted in a high pitched nasal voice, "You have to look at my baby! I mean look at him now!" Her loud shouting and her rudeness indicated no respect for the clients already waiting to see me or, for that matter, for me.

I was amazed at this loud, demanding woman. Composing myself I said, in the most professional tone I could muster, "Is this an emergency?" I waited for her to hear what I had to say and then continued, "If not, these people are ahead of you."

I had never seen this person before. I glanced out the window toward the parking lot at their car. It had Ohio license tags. Standing beside the car a younger man was holding a baby's bassinet that was covered with a baby blanket. This bassinet obviously held some sort of an animal. I didn't try to second guess this case, or even speculate what kind of a pet was in the baby carrier, but I did have a gut feeling this was going to be an interesting experience.

Never bothering to answer me, the woman turned back to the door and yelled for the man to come in.

By this time I was completely frustrated. What composure I had was lost! My clients in the waiting room couldn't help but overhear the entire conversation. I am sure they wondered what was to come next. One of them, an old friend, looked at me and said, "Doc, what do you suppose is in that basket?"

The man came in with the bassinet and set it on my examination table. The woman, talking so fast she was hard to understand, jabbered that the veterinarian in her town was no good. She kept it up and said he was mean, hateful and she was thinking about suing him!

Now I was definitely on the defensive, and only after seeing what was in that baby bed, did I consent to try and help this loud, demanding person.

Tears streaming down her face, the lady pulled the cover away from her ward and there was a tiny chimpanzee, pale, obviously dehydrated and seemingly near death. The chimp's diaper was soaked with watery fecal matter. The odor was terrible. It didn't take a circus doctor to realize this animal had an intestinal problem and was critically ill. I questioned her about how long the chimp had been sick and what she had done for it.

Then the lady shouted at me in a voice loud enough to be heard down the street, "I don't believe in medicine, I don't believe in doctors." She picked the sick animal up and held it in her arms, gently rocking it back and forth like a small baby. Then she said, her whole attitude changing to a gentle approach, "Doctor, do something."

My better judgment told me to ask her to leave. My compassion for that poor baby chimp challenged me. I asked her to listen to me and I would tell her what we basically had to do if we were going to save the animal's life.

"Intravenous fluids are first," I said. "Then we are going to try and find out what is wrong. It may be parasites or a bacterial infection."

Before I could say another word she yelled at me again, "You're just like them other vets. Tellin' me my baby has worms." She looked me straight in the eye and added, "Mister, you are wrong!"

By this time the waiting room people had focused all of their attention on the conversation and they heard every word that transpired between us.

Now I was angry, tired of being verbally abused and tired of being threatened. I never hesitated and in a very demanding voice said, "You and your man friend and your chimpanzee get out of here and do not come back." The crowd in the waiting room rumbled what I hoped was their approval. Then I took another look at that poor sick chimp. It really needed some medical attention. I calmed down and finally suggested we look at the animal.

My demanding tone of voice made her believe I was not to be intimidated. Finally, looking at the man, who I later found out was her mentally retarded son, she told him it was all right for me to look at the sick one.

A complete examination revealed severe dehydration and I started an IV at once. I suggested we put her animal in the hospital for continued treatment. With a louder voice than before, she yelled at me, "No—I can take better care of him than you can." I did not argue the point. We moved this woman, her son and the chimp with the IV going into his arm, into another room and took care of the other clients. Everyone I saw that evening made me promise to let them know how the case turned out.

The IV helped. The little dehydrated chimp opened his eyes and if a monkey could smile, he smiled at me. I dispensed some liquid intestinal antibiotics, an anti-diarrhea medicine and sent her back to Ohio with instructions to come back the next evening.

This woman, in my opinion, like her son, was not mentally straight. She said she would be back. I saw her again the next day and the next and the next! Between visits she called me several times on the telephone asking me questions and talking about how awful her hometown veterinarian was. I made every effort to applaud her doctor, who was my good friend, Dr. Owen Karr, and tried my best to get her to take her animals back to him.

The sick chimpanzee responded well to my treatment, but when I tried to get her to make some management changes, such as a better diet and better sanitation, she screamed at me, and for the first time using profanity, "You're no damned good, you are just like the rest of 'em, I may even sue you!"

In the meantime I had talked to my friend Dr. Karr and he assured me this was her routine with every veterinarian in the area. She threatened a lawsuit to each and every one, but none ever materialized. He assured me, if she was true to form, she would never be back. Before we hung up the telephone, he asked me, "Did she pay you?"

"Every penny," I said.

"You can thank me for that," Karr said, "Because I told her you were a high class circus doctor and a real expert with chimpanzees. I made it clear to her that you wouldn't even talk to her unless she had the money up front! Matter of fact, she owes all of us in our town money!"

After the conversation was finished, I gave some thought to this lady, her retarded grown son and her sick animal. It had been a trying experience but my reward was getting that monkey well plus getting paid! This case was closed. Dr. Karr was right, we never heard from her again!

In the never ho-hum world of my kind of veterinary medicine, surprises were part of every day. I took the unusual in stride.

There were pleasant times too. Early one nice spring morning I had just finished delivering a calf at the McGlothlin dairy farm. I was cleaning my equipment and putting it away in the car when Mrs. McGlothlin came to the barn and told me I was to call my office when I was through.

The house was just across the road from the dairy and I walked around to the kitchen door to make my call. Mrs. McGlothlin, a jewel of a lady, said, "Doc, your office help said something about an elephant they want you to look at." Everybody knew about my exotic animal work so it didn't surprise them when I got the phone call. "Don't suppose it's trying to have a calf too, do you." She laughed and poured me a cup of coffee while I dialed the office.

Charlie Allen, who stayed for a while at my clinic with his bears and zebra, was in Huntington, West Virginia, ready to play a Shrine

Circus date at the local amusement park.

Charlie and I said our hellos. I inquired about his family's health; he asked about mine. The greetings were over and Charlie told me he had an elephant rented for the season and it had a big swollen place on its hip. He said it was an unsightly place and was afraid that the audience response wouldn't be favorable looking at this. "Doc, can you come up and take a look at it for me?"

I told him I would be there within the hour and to try and have some help in case we needed to restrain his "bull."

I stopped by our house and picked up my wife, knowing she would be glad to see the Allens again. We drove on to the park. The elephant had a big abscess on its hip, probably where it had backed into a nail or laid on a big splintered chunk of wood.

Charlie held the elephant's tail out of the way, his helper got the bull's attention with the bull hook and a big pile of fresh hay. I carefully examined the grapefruit sized lump. It was indeed an abscess and I made quick work of opening and draining it. I packed the cavernous hole with medicated gauze, left instructions with Charlie and told him and his wife, Beverly, that we would see them at the circus the next day.

I drove away from the barn where the Allens had their circus stock and stopped at the amusement park office to use the phone and check in with my office. Harry Nudd, one of the owners of the park, told me he was just ready to call me and wanted to know if I could come up and shoot some bears with my tranquilizer gun. He wanted to move these bears to a new compound he built earlier that year while the bears were in the dens with their newborn cubs. Now the cubs were big enough to go outside and it was time for the move. I agreed to come early the next morning before the park opened.

I was at the park by eight o'clock. Nudd and his helpers were ready for me. The tranquilizer gun was new in those days and I showed it to everybody and explained how it worked. I also explained the drug I intended using was very short acting and the men would have to work quickly before the effect of the drug wore off.

I loaded the gun with my dart of medicine and Harry coaxed the first bear out of the den with some food. Carefully I took aim and pulled the trigger. The dart hit home with very little discomfort to the bruin. We waited for it to take effect. We waited five minutes. By now the bear should be getting sleepy. Ten minutes later it was obvious the dose had little or no effect. I fixed another dart. This dart had a longer needle because I suspected that the heavy layer of fat carried by a bear might prevent my medicine from working. I pulled the trigger again. This time a little vocal bear objection, like a snarl! The results were the same. It was obvious that my method was not going to work.

Harry Nudd thanked me for my time and told his men to come in the cage with him. Each one grabbed a bear—there were three of them—and manually forced each animal out, across the sidewalk into their new den! Harry got the job done—his way. After discussing what went wrong with the gun business, we decided that my concern not to overdose the bears had been the shortcoming. I put the gun away and I never used it again.

From Harry Nudd's amusement park office I drove back past Charlie Allen's. My wife and I waved as we went by. Then I drove on to my next farm visit to vaccinate some hogs.

I considered these situations as pure business in my practice, albeit my house calls and some cases differed from most veterinarian's.

Not every memorable episode was directly related to sick animals. The human interest side of my career occasionally showed up in one way or another.

On a more somber note—I was up on Bolt's Fork where I had just finished vaccinating some calves for Bang's disease. I was taking my time driving along the country road when a man I knew flagged me down and asked me, "If'n you get to town will you call me an ambulance? Maw's sick, Doc, I think she's havin' one of her heart spells. Doc, if'n ya don't mind, hurry. She's in bad shape."

Lester Holbrook was this fellow's name and I said, "Lester, I'll just call my office on my car radio and have Stormy call the ambulance—we'll have that ambulance here in no time at all." I thought a minute and not knowing if it was proper or not, I said, "Is there any way my knowledge can help your mother?"

"Nope, Doc, thanks, we give her pills and I think she'll be OK, if we kin get her to the hospital. You just don't know how much I appreciate you-ah-calling on your radio for us."

I told him I was glad to help and made him promise he would let me know about his mother's condition. In about a week I got a little note, written in pencil on a piece of yellow tablet paper, that "Maw" Holbrook was doing fine. It's things like this that make me proud that I can sometimes help in other ways besides doctoring a cow or a horse.

There was one more—not so bizarre, but I thought at the time a little unusual, incident that perhaps can be included in the nature of my wonderful Kentucky hill country.

Just before Christmas on a cold, rainy day, my first country call was in the next county to conduct an autopsy on a cow that had died the night before. The onset of death was sudden and the cause of the cow's death was unknown. Mr. Walker, the farmer, suspected food poisoning, but on my suggestion we did not rule out an infectious disease. Walker owned several head of cattle and was worried that he would lose more if the real cause of death wasn't determined.

I left my office in a cloudburst of rain and followed the main paved highway to a turnoff on a graveled county road. I followed this road to another turnoff, this one partly through a creek bed that was running six inches deep because of the downpour of rain. As I drove along through the water, I glanced out of the car window and saw four people up on a hilltop to my left. The thought immediately went through my mind that the dead cow was up there. I pictured myself climbing that steep hill and doing an autopsy in this awful storm. I finally got to the Walker's and drove up on a piece of high ground and parked behind their small frame house. This house obviously had started like so many old farmhouses as a single log building then as time went by, an identical unit was added. This made a house with a center hall between two large rooms. A porch along the entire back side of house seemed to tie it all together. Most early farmhouses in our country seemed to evolve this way. More additions were added as more space was needed. Eventually they were covered with siding.

I got out of my car just as a lady came out the back door to draw a bucket of water from a covered well at the edge of the porch. "Good morning, Mrs. Walker, Merry Christmas."

"I thank you, Doctor, but it ain't a very merry Christmas here," she hesitated then went on, "Just after Thanksgiving Uncle Charles passed away and now, Aunt Minnie is a layin' a corpse!"

I couldn't help seeing through the open back door of this house. I saw the dead lady laid out on a house door that was supported on two sawhorses. She was covered with a beautiful homemade quilt. A single vase of artificial flowers sat by the foot of her final bed.

"I offer my sincere regrets, Mrs. Walker—I am so sorry for you." And then it dawned on me, that the men on top of the hill were digging a grave for Aunt Minnie! Then I asked, "Where is the cow and where is the cow feed?"

As she turned to go back into the house, she said, "The cow is out in the barn and the feed is in the smokehouse."

I thanked her and walked a short distance to the smokehouse and opened the door and walked in. Sure enough there was a big bin full of commercial cow feed. It looked OK to me. Then as I turned around to go look at the cow, I saw a homemade coffin standing on its end in one corner of the smokehouse. Some of the boards still had bark on them. So now the whole picture came to me.

I examined the dead animal and reported my findings to Mrs. Walker and drove back to town through even heavier rain. That night when I got home I told Mary Helen about my strange sad visit that morning. We both realized this lady was not embalmed, but that is no infraction of the rules in Kentucky. We also realized she wouldn't rest in a fancy casket. She was simply returned to the ground—truly, dust to dust.

The next day we checked the obituary column in our local paper and there it was, a short notice saying, in essence, that Mrs. Walker of Sand Suck, Greenup County, passed away. The service would be conducted by the minister from Old Steam Church. And burial would be in the family cemetery on Culp Creek. Ways as old as the ages were still being practiced in our Kentucky Hill Country.

Whoever said, "All the glitter, excitement, mystique and magic is at the circus?"

THE CONCERT

In the old time tented circus days, most circuses held a concert. This was circus jargon for an additional performance given in the Big Top for an extra fee after the main show was over. It usually was a wild west show or a novelty show. As a rule, the performers did not play in the main show. This exhibition was also sometimes called, "The After Show." It was the last gasp and when it was finished, the circus activities were over until the next scheduled performance. It was also the last chance for the management to get some of the local money. Show folks say, at this point, and using another circus term, the show is, "all out and all over."

Now it's time for my concert.

The veterinary practice has changed. There are many new concepts of veterinary medicine and much new knowledge. Some of the diseases we considered years ago as untreatable such as twisted stomachs in cattle, certain bacterial diseases of dogs and cats, and heart worms in dogs are now routinely treated and end with good results. Many new treatments and diagnostic aids have changed the entire scene from my time. Veterinary medicine has changed a lot over the years—all of it for the good.

Exotic animal medicine has made great strides, far from the hit-and-miss techniques that Dr. Henderson taught me and I practiced in most of the circus tents and buildings in our land. They weren't wrong and at the time, were the best ideas we had. As new technology developed, Henderson and I grabbed it quickly and both of us used it trying to better our type of veterinary care. Perhaps one of the greatest major developments was the newer, safer, easier-to-use anesthetics. The time of the big cats sleeping for days is over. There is no more getting a rope around a lion's or tiger's leg and pulling it through the bars and trying to inject a drug to put it to sleep. Instead, there are new antibiotics and pharmaceuticals that were developed by animal research.

In the early days, Dr. J.Y. Henderson was the authority. Thankfully he took me under his wing and taught me most of what I know about the circus animals. Together we developed some new techniques that were quickly picked up by our followers.

Today exotic animal medicine is part of the college curriculum and the newly capped DVM has at least been exposed to the need for this kind of medicine.

All of the zoos have on staff or on call veterinarians who have been trained to do their work. They have contributed much to today's exotic animal science.

As the years went by, I employed most of the boys in the neighborhood for one thing or another. They cut grass, cleaned out the barn, built fences, painted and once in a while they helped with little jobs in the clinic.

Gary Duncan was one of these neighborhood kids and he insisted he was going to someday be a veterinarian, "Just like you, Doc." He persisted with his goal and I respected him so much for that—maybe remembering my ambition and my desire to be an animal doctor. I guess I was to him what Doctor Karr had been to me—an inspiration.

I was proud of him and was his voucher and supporter when it came time for him to enter the university. He was a good student and dedicated to quality veterinary medicine. He worked for me in the summer and when the time came he did part of his internship in my clinic.

While he was with me it became obvious he would someday return to Ashland and, it was a foregone conclusion he would eventually own the clinic. After graduation he spent some time in a surgical internship. After that he operated an emergency clinic for a veterinary group in Cincinnati. He gained valuable experience and if he was to make any mistakes, I told him, "to make them before you come back to Kentucky."

Late in the fall some years ago, Gary Duncan, DVM, called me and said he was ready to assume my practice and my clinic if I was still willing. We closed the deal on the last day of December, 1986. I stayed for a few months during the ownership transition and then I left. After thirty-seven years, I was finally unemployed!

Dr. Duncan retained the name, the Martin Veterinary Clinic, and with it, its reputation. Perhaps this is some monument to me and my career and I am grateful for that. The practice has grown and serves only small animals now and is truly a state of the art facility. There are presently nine or ten veterinarians in our town and Gary does the most work by far.

I have had opportunity to watch the new-style vet in action myself. Mary Helen and I have an old black cat. She was a feral cat, a creature of the woods. One day the cat came walking up one of our fencelines leading a small kitten. My wife and I watched her as she very cautiously, with every step, checked to be sure it was safe. The next day she repeated the same pattern only this time she had three kittens with her! I suggested to Mary Helen to put some food out for the cat. I also suggested maybe she could tame her and since she was such a pretty cat we could enjoy her as our own.

It took two years to get the cat to where Mary Helen could even touch her. In the meantime she had two or three litters of kittens in our big barn. The kittens were as wild as she was and as they grew up, they left and went their own wild ways. In time, after my wife had made her feel at home, I caught the cat and spayed her. She was an adult cat then and we have had her twelve or thirteen years. Heaven knows how old she really is but she is still apprehensive, aware of strangers and keeps her old wild instinct of preservation. It has only been in the last year or so I could pet her or pick her up. We named her Tara.

Some time ago Tara got sick and I took her to Dr. Duncan. This was a new experience to me. Now I was the client, across the table from the doctor, grasping for some help and hope for my animal. Gary diagnosed her as having feline immune deficiency syndrome—a viral disease that I had never heard of in my time. He treated her and I brought her back to Jomar for her final days.

When I attended Ohio State University Veterinary College, I only knew of three lady veterinarians. Today the ladies represent sixty percent of the entire profession. Most of these serve the small animals but some are bound and determined to be large animal practitioners. I know they are well trained and determined but yet I can't bring myself to believe that they can endure the obvious that goes with large animal medicine. The physical hurts, the strength sometimes needed for the services and the unbelievable long hours are still there. But yet they do it and are successful. I applaud them for what they do.

After Dr. Duncan assumed ownership of the Martin Veterinary Clinic, I retired to a legacy of memories of those wonderful years. My best memories are of the friends I have made and the people who have been part of my life here in the hills of Kentucky and under the canvas Big Tops of the circus. I shared their joys at birthings—both human and my kind—and shared their sorrows with them as they or their animals passed away. I have seen the parents with their little children bring me their puppies or their kittens for my services. Then I saw those children grow up and it was their turn to bring their little ones and their pets to me.

An old adage says, "What goes around, comes around." That is certainly true. After I retired from active practice of veterinary medicine, I went back to my other profession—aviation. Today I am again a professional airplane pilot—albeit older than most. I enjoy teaching young people to share with me the freedom of flight that has enthralled me over these last fifty years. I still remember flying over Arabia and looking down at the man leading his camel up the hospital ramp so the doctor could tend to its Asiatic illness. I remember landing my airplane in a farmer's field to make my house call! At one of my Bluegrass horse farms I routinely flew into a tobacco patch airstrip to treat their show horses. I'll never forget flying to the circus in the mountain town and that wild car ride down the highway to the circus grounds. My insurance friend, Charles, is still around and we still talk about what he called ". . . our adventures." He was right, they were adventures.

So call this my concert—the after show, if you will. I still consult and discuss cases with the circus people and count as my very true friends literally hundreds of performers and ex-performers. There is never a day at least one of them doesn't call for advice or just to talk or, as they say in circus talk, "to cut up jackpots."

But before "its all out and all over," I want to bring up topics that I am still questioned about.

Whether I was on the road with a show or working in the clinic I was often asked the same two questions. The first one is "Doctor, isn't the life of circus veterinarian terrifically exciting?"

My stock answer is "No, most of the work is preventive medicine with a lot of standing around hoping nothing bad will happen."

The other question—the one I am most often asked is, "What are the most dangerous animals you work with?" I never hesitate and I tell the questioner these animals are the bear and the chimpanzee. The bear, because he doesn't retract his claws and uses what he has like a hand full of knives. If you try to confine him, he just rolls up in a ball and uses his nasty mouth full of teeth and his razor sharp claws. He fights you—he is a killing machine.

I let that sink in for a minute and then talk about the next meanest—the chimpanzee. The chimp in a sense has four hands and a mouth full of very big sharp teeth. A mean chimp out of control is capable of breaking your leg with one bite or biting off your hand or finger in a flash. He is strong of arm and can do you harm with those pendulous arms and hands. As cute as he is—he is dangerous.

And then I add, "You should have asked, what animal is the most likely to hurt you? Is it the lion or the tiger? No, because we keep them caged and use every precaution in the world to avoid getting hurt by them. Is it the elephant? No, because here again we safeguard against these big animals with every precaution we have to confine them and protect the public." I let this soak in for a minute and then finally and emphatically I add, "It is the animal we take for granted. We accept him as part of our heritage and some of us as part of our everyday lives. We get careless, we get complacent—and then it happens. The animal that is most likely to hurt you is—the horse!"

The horse—the critter that started it all for me—is still around and when I see one I am indebted to it for the part its kind played in my career and my life. Perhaps that animal—or an animal of some other species—will inspire some other young person to pursue a career as a Doctor of Veterinary Medicine.

My determination to become a veterinarian became a reality and my passion for animals and their welfare became an obsession. It is not a field of endeavor for everybody, but for those dedicated few, I think it is a wonderful profession.

If someone does follow in my footsteps, I can assure him, or her, of a very rewarding life. Maybe he or she will never get a phone call from someone like Pat Anthony saying, "Doc, my tiger's got an itch." Chances are he or she will never doctor a lion or tiger or a bear. It is not likely a phone call will come from some owner to put a mule to sleep so he could nail a shoe, "on the son-of-a-bitch." But I am sure they will have their stories to tell about the usual and unusual things that happened in their careers. One thing is certain, they will have the satisfaction, as I did, of being part of and serving a glorious profession.

In the circus they often use one more term, "Finale." It means it's finished.

EPILOGUE

I owe so much to so many people who inspired this book. Everyone mentioned is real and each and every one of them has my warmest thanks for being part of my life. I have used real names and places where I could. If I have offended anybody, it was not intentional because I respect all of them.

I am also indebted to a very few special people who were responsible for my career, and its consequences, and to those who inspired me to write this book. For my gratitude for their part in my life, I sincerely dedicate my story to them.

In memory of

Owen M. Karr, DVM   Portsmouth, Ohio

My idol, my voucher, my friend and a great teacher. It was Dr. Karr who inspired me to become a Doctor Of Veterinary Medicine.

In memory of

J.Y. Henderson, DVM   Sarasota , Florida

Chief veterinarian for Ringling Bros. and Barnum & Bailey Circus who, along with his family, became the greatest friend we ever had. Dr. Henderson put the sawdust in my veins. Knowledge about his work led me to follow in his footsteps as a circus doctor.

In Memory of

Jesse Stuart　　　　　　Greenup, Kentucky

Poet Laureate of Kentucky, author of many books—including: *The Man with the Bull Tongue Plow*, and *Taps for Private Tussey*. He was a Kentucky farmer, one of my high school teachers and a very good friend. Jesse Stuart insisted that someday I tell about my experiences in the Highlands, with the circus and on the farmlands of Kentucky.

With sincere gratitude to

Billy C. Clark　　　　　　Catlettsburg, Kentucky

Author of *A Long Row to Hoe, The Trail of the Hunter's Horn, The Champion of Sourwood Mountain*, and many other stories. Along with Jesse Stuart, Billy inspired me to tell some of my stories.

Billy Clark is the founder and editor of *Virginia Writing* at Longwood College in Farmville, Virginia. He is a dear friend with whom I share many fond memories of my early days as a Kentucky hill country veterinarian.

All of my love, appreciation and affection to

Mary Helen Feyler Martin

My wife worked side by side with me through the years in college while I was learning, through the good years and the hard times of those early years in practice and stood by me when the pitfalls were the deepest. Thanks always, Mary Helen, for this and for bearing and rearing our daughter.

Gee Gee Engesser

Gee Gee is a classy, talented performer, a very capable animal handler and a devoted mother.

I am extremely proud that you, the First Lady of the American Circus, have honored me with praise and flattery in your introduction to this book. My gratitude will be never-ending.

Teresa Lynn Martin Klaiber

Apple of a father's eye, horsewoman, mother of our grandchildren and daddy's biggest booster.

My very sincere thanks to my clients and friends who owned the cows, the horses, the cats and dogs, lions, tigers, elephants, bears, zebras, reptiles, llamas and other exotic and not so exotic animals that paid the bills and created and cemented life long friendships. Without you, it would never have happened.

And finally, thanks to The Horse.

The critter which started it all!

THE EVOLUTION OF EXOTIC ANIMAL MEDICINE

Veterinary medicine for the exotic species has come a long way since the early years of the traveling circuses and menageries.

Today you will not see a horse destroyed because of a repairable fracture, nor will you see wounds cauterized with red hot irons to promote healing. Restraint by brute force is no longer necessary thanks to modern day tranquilizers and anesthetics. Complicated lifesaving surgical procedures are routinely performed. Disease prevention and control is now a reality, because of modern day vaccinations and medical knowledge.

In the early 1940s, Ringling Bros. and Barnum & Bailey Circus employed Dr. J.Y. Henderson, and for a time, Dr. William Higgins, to care for the health of their large collection of valuable animals. Eventually, comparing the exotics to their counterparts in domestic medicine, Dr. Henderson developed techniques that proved successful with the exotic animals. He was recognized as an authority in this field. Henderson befriended the author and urged him to follow this line of work. These doctors today are considered the pioneers of circus medicine as we know it today.

In time a foundation of knowledge began to build. The circus veterinarian's expertise was compared to the findings of the zoo doctors such as Clinton Grey, National Zoo in Washington, D.C. and Lee Simmons, Henry Doorley Zoo in Omaha. Scientists began new research. The pharmaceutical companies developed new drugs and well-known animal trainers told their secrets. U.S. Seale, Ph.D., a medical researcher, can be thanked for his research in blood chemistries with the Ringing circus animals. The veterinary colleges also recognized the need for trained doctors in exotic medicine and added courses for interested students, and today the interest in this field of veterinary medicine is at an all-time high.

Sixty years have passed since the day Clyde Beatty poured iodine on his wounded tiger. That kind of treatment is in the past. Zoos and circuses have flourished, and most have veterinarians on staff or on call. Ringling Bros. and Barnum & Bailey Circus, the pioneer in employing veterinarians, again has its own full-time veterinarian, Dr. Richard Hauck. Carson & Barnes Circus in Hugo, Oklahoma, considers their local veterinarian one of their staff. Others, like the author, act as consultants for circuses and privately owned animal acts. This type of work has become routine; the future looks bright for exotic medicine.